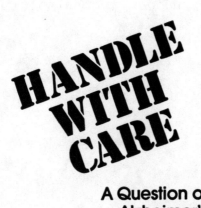

HANDLE WITH CARE

**A Question of
Alzheimer's**

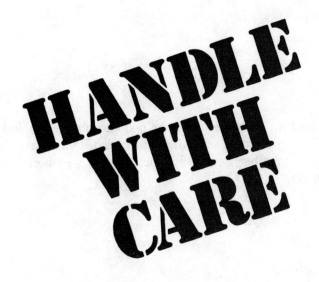

A Question of
Alzheimer's

Dorothy S. Brown

Prometheus Books
700 East Amherst Street, Buffalo, New   York 14215
In cooperation with
Potentials Development for Health & Aging Services, Inc.
775 Main Street, Suite 321, Buffalo, New   York 14203

852391

To

my mother and all the people who helped care for her, including Michael, Sarah, David, and Jeremiah, also Rachel, who is
too young to remember her, and Rebecca, who was born too
late to know her.

Published 1984 by Prometheus Books in cooperation with Potentials Development for Health & Aging Services Inc.

Library of Congress Card Catalog No. 84-61253
ISBN: 087975-271-8 (cloth)
    0-9392910-47-5 (paper)

Contents

PREFACE

My first reactions to my mother's condition were shock, despair, and bewilderment. I was shocked at the amount of weight she had lost in the ten months since I had last seen her and at her seriously impaired mind. I felt despair when I recognized the extent of her dependence on me and the sudden responsibility for which I was unprepared. I was bewildered by her confusion.

Shock is generally temporary and I recovered from it. My despair decreased and disappeared eventually, when I realized that although I was responsible for Mother's welfare and had to make decisions, friends and relatives were willing to help me—and her. All of us tried in as many ways as we could think of to make life less unpleasant for her, and occasionally we succeeded.

I am still bewildered. I do not know exactly what went wrong in her brain, but I believe that if her condition had become obvious in 1980 instead of 1970, it would have been diagnosed as Alzheimer's disease. Since her death, I have had time to read about others with similar symptoms and about current research in disorders of the brain. My reading has served as a background for the focal point of this book, which is primarily about my mother's illness.

Just as friends helped my mother and me when she was alive, I have had the help and encouragement of many friends in writing this book. I want to thank especially Maureen Faulkner, emeritus professor of English, who read each chapter carefully as soon as it was completed and offered invaluable suggestions. I am indebted to John Runda, Ph.D., and Audrey Runda, R.N., owners and managers of a nursing home, to Faith Birznieks, a Claims Representative for the Social Security Administration, and to Harold Brody, M.D., Ph.D., of the State University of New York at Buffalo, past president of the Gerontological Society, for reading the parts of the manuscript in which they have expertise. I accept full responsibility for any mistakes, misinterpretations, or misleading statements. I am also indebted to other friends, too numerous to mention, who called my attention to recent books, magazine articles, newspaper stories, and television programs related to the care of dementia patients.

In writing this book I have been deliberately vague about the location of events described and the names of most of the people mentioned. When writing of hypothetical patients I have used feminine pronouns throughout, because women make up the majority of people suffering from Alzheimer's disease and because the book is about my mother.

Although my purpose has been to show how I dealt with my mother's illness, I hope that this book will be helpful to others who care for fathers, husbands, wives, and other relatives, as well as for mothers.

CHAPTER I

Early Warning Signals

My mother was a very clever woman. Before the days of adding machines when grocery clerks wrote down each item by hand and then totaled the cost, she would stand on the customer side of the counter reading the prices upside down, and arrive at the correct sum before the clerk had finished adding. As far as I know she never lost this skill, though in the days of computers and adding machines she had fewer occasions to use it.

She was an excellent bridge player too. I suspect that she added up all scores, as she did the items on sales slips, upside down or sideways—unless, of course, she was keeping score herself. Her partners and her opponents were all serious about the game, and occasionally there were words exchanged, but they continued to play together until Mother and one of her friends had some kind of disagreement at a bridge tournament. It must have been trivial as the friend never learned what she had done or said to offend my mother. Partly as a result of this incident Mother stopped playing bridge.

I saw nothing unusual in Mother's behavior toward her friend; she had always been easily offended and slow to forgive an offense.

She did not give up bridge entirely. Instead, she arranged with a hotel to be the hostess for Friday night bridge games. She set up the tables (it was all duplicate, of course, with each table having identical hands dealt), introduced herself to the guests and the guests to each other, greeted people, chatted with them, and saw that everything ran smoothly. She was good at that sort of thing.

It was typical of her to find a way to keep in touch with the bridge world, even though she no longer played. My mother had always been resourceful.

At this time she was in her late sixties and as lively and active as she had ever been. She had retired from teaching at sixty-five, and for two years after that had done substitute teaching, taking an intense interest in whatever subject she happened to be teaching for the day. Later, when she had to give up substitute work because of age regulations, she began working a few hours a day at a private high school where she kept attendance records, collected lunch money, and did some bookkeeping. She continued to be active in her church, taking pride in arranging the flowers for the altar each Sunday. She still drove her car.

One day when she was driving in heavy traffic her car was hit by another car. The damage was slight but Mother had to go to court. Even though the judge ruled that the accident was not her fault, he told her that he would have to take her license away because of her age. This upset my mother so much that she became almost hysterical. By enlisting the aid of her pastor and other friends, she persuaded the judge to let her keep her license until I returned from a prolonged trip. "When my daughter comes back," she told the judge, "she can drive for me. But until then I *have* to drive my car." Her most urgent need was to go to a florist's shop once a week to buy flowers to decorate the church, and many of the church members would gladly have taken her. But she did not want to depend on others. She had always been independent.

When I returned I went with her to see the judge, who let her retain her license after I told him that her age had not, I was sure, affected her driving. But the incident seemed to take away some of her self-confidence, and partly as a result of it she decided to stop working. She also talked of going for a long visit with her sisters the following fall.

She told many people of her plans: the teachers, other workers at the school, and her friends. The one person whom she did not tell, however, was her principal, Mr. Larsen. I urged her to tell him so that he could begin looking for someone to replace her, but she made excuses. At first she said that he had so much on his mind, so many things to worry about, that it would upset him to learn that one of his employees was not returning in the fall. Later she remarked sulkily that he never showed any consideration for *her* and she saw no reason for telling him of her plans. By this time Mr. Larsen had heard rumors from his staff that Mother was not returning the following year. Summer came, however, the school year was over, and she still had not notified him.

I could understand her reluctance; she had worked all of her life, having started as a clerk in a department store on Saturdays when she was twelve years old. She enjoyed working, whether in a business firm or in a school. I had never known her to have a job that she did not like. So giving up this last job must have been, for her, like giving up a very important part of her life. No wonder she was reluctant to submit her resignation.

Finally, Mr. Larsen called me and asked if I knew what my mother's plans were. I told him that she did not plan to return, and added that she could not seem to bring herself to resign. Mr. Larsen, a young man of great understanding, proposed a strategy.

Mother's office was across the hall from the principal's office. She still went to it once or twice a week, bringing home a few papers and other materials each time, prolonging the moving out process as long as possible. Mr. Larsen asked me to call him at his home, which was near the school, the next time Mother set out for her office, so that he could be in his own office when she arrived. He would then drop in on her for a casual chat and try to get her to tell him of her plans.

The strategy worked well. The next time Mother started out for her office I notified Mr. Larsen. I do not know what they said to each other, but when Mother came home she was in an exuberant mood and rather proud of herself. "I told Mr. Larsen that I'm not going to work next fall," she reported cheerfully, "and he took it very well. I think I managed the conversation with him rather nicely."

Since Mother planned to be away for several months, she rented her home for the semester. She planned to visit her sisters from September until after Christmas; she was to look at apartments near them, with the idea of possibly making a permanent move. I planned to take an early retirement at age fifty-five, and to settle somewhere in the East nearer where our relatives lived, but not in the same city. Mother and I both felt that she would be happier with her sisters and other relatives, in a city where she already knew many people, than with me in a strange place.

I learned later from the relatives whom she visited that she showed little or no interest in looking at apartments. In fact, they said, she showed little interest in doing anything. On previous visits she had been eager to plan and prepare meals, entertain friends, help with sewing and other chores. On this visit she never offered to do anything except to wrap Christmas presents and it took her hours, one of my cousins told me later, to wrap one present.

That did not surprise me. She had always been meticulous about wrapping presents; in fact, I have never known anyone who wrapped them as neatly or attractively.

When she returned after Christmas, she refused to consider moving out of her house either to live near her sisters or to go to a retirement home, a possibility which she had considered with some enthusiasm a few years earlier. "I'm not ready for that yet," she now insisted.

Meanwhile, my own arrangements for retiring and taking another position had been completed. Mother argued that I could not begin collecting my state retirement pension until I was sixty-five, even though I explained carefully to her that the State Retirement Office had told me that it could be collected at age fifty-five. I knew that she was reluctant for me to leave and I was not comfortable about leaving her alone, but she seemed in good health, she had many friends, and she certainly had the right to live where she pleased.

Her insistence that I would have to wait ten years before collecting my retirement income was motivated, I began to suspect, by her reluctance to see me leave. She was wrong about the retirement; whether I was right or wrong about her motive I still do not know.

After I left, Mother began writing me long letters, mostly about her problems with arthritis. It was not like her to complain of her health; she had always stayed well. I did not consider her problems serious. Believing that she had not wanted me to leave, I thought that she was exaggerating the arthritis pains, perhaps hoping that I would return. Or, I thought with some resentment and a slight touch of guilt, she might have been trying to get even with me for leaving. At any rate, I could not turn back; I had retired from my job, sold my house, and committed myself to a new position several thousand miles away.

Ironically, after I left, my daughter returned to attend the university where I had been teaching. She had been living in a city not far from my new place of employment, and I had looked forward to being somewhat closer to her. Although I was disappointed that she would still be so far away from me, I was relieved that someone in the family would be near Mother.

At first my daughter stayed with friends, but when she realized that her grandmother's health was failing she moved in with her. The most obvious symptom of Mother's failing health was weight loss. She seemed to have no appetite.

My daughter would go grocery shopping and bring back whatever she had been asked to buy, and more. Then Mother would telephone her friends and complain that there was nothing in the house to eat, though the freezer compartment of the refrigerator was bulging with food and the shelves were lined with canned goods. But Mother would not cook, nor would she eat what her granddaughter prepared. Some of her friends tried taking her out to lunch and urging her to eat, but she merely picked at her food. Other friends took her cake and cookies and helped her prepare a pot of tea, but afternoon tea parties are not an adequate substitute for a well-balanced diet. Naturally she lost weight rapidly.

My daughter wrote me all this, adding that she thought her grandmother was dying. I continued to explain away the warning signs. *She is exaggerating,* I thought. *They are just having problems with each other.* My mother, who liked to wait on people, had always got along better with her grandson who liked to be waited on, than with her granddaughter who was more independent.

But my daughter was not exaggerating. On April 1, 1970, I received a telegram from a friend, telling me that something would have to be done about Mother, and asking me to call him. While I was waiting for the evening rates and, I thought, giving our friend time to get home from work, he telephoned me.

He was obviously upset, not only about my mother's condition but also about the fact that I had not yet called him. He told me that Mother was seriously ill and that someone would have to come for her immediately, but he was vague about the nature of her illness. We agreed that the best course would be to enlist the aid of one of her sisters. After I had several telephone conversations with various family members, it was decided that the youngest sister would go, accompanied by her husband, a retired airline employee. They could therefore travel for half fare, which was a tremendous help.

Upon their arrival they found that Mother had not only lost weight, she was also greatly confused. Our friend told them that he had realized something was wrong when Mother asked him to help with her taxes and then insisted that she was not receiving Social Security. He knew that she was, and he later found several unopened checks in the house. That was when he decided to call me.

All this time Mother was writing me perfectly lucid and sometimes even witty letters. She had stopped complaining about her arthritis, and instead was expressing concern about all the people in the house: her sister, her brother-in-law, her granddaughter. She did not seem to realize that they were there to help her and she felt that she had to take care of them. That seemed to me perfectly normal behavior for my mother. It was her house; she should be in charge. I did not believe that anything was seriously wrong, though I did think it an excellent idea for her to sell her home and move closer to our relatives.

My aunt and uncle had arrived in the middle of April and Mother's house was sold May 1. The next step was for movers to pack her possessions, of which she had many. Mother directed their work, all the time protesting that she was not going to leave. Surprisingly, she did a more than creditable job of selecting the items to be packed and shipped.

Meanwhile, my uncle wrote that he had taken over Mother's checkbook and balanced it, as she seemed incapable.

My mother incapable of balancing a checkbook? Why, she used to be an accountant, and she had taught business math in high school for years. I was certain that her problems, whatever they were, were only temporary, and that once she was with her family she would be all right.

My aunt and uncle took her to their home to live until I could meet her there and decide what to do. As soon as the spring term was over I drove to their home, a distance of about five hundred miles. I was apprehensive but still certain that this would not be a problem I couldn't handle. My aunt had suggested that I consider putting her in a nursing home. It seemed a reasonable solution, but I thought it possible that Mother could settle down in a comfortable apartment near her sisters, and that with a little outside help she could still live alone.

My uncle had brought with him a stack of Mother's unpaid bills, and soon after I arrived he gave them to me to take care of. I set up a card table, spread some of the bills in front of Mother and gave her one of her checkbooks. I thought that if I re-created the atmosphere in which she used to write checks, everything would be normal.

It wasn't. She stared at the checkbook. Finally she asked, "What day is today?" I told her the date, but she did not write it down. Instead, she asked again, "What day is today?" She continued to stare at the check. After about fifteen minutes, during which time she continued to ask the same question and to stare blankly at her checkbook, I gave up and put the bills away.

Getting the bills paid was not a problem as for years my name had been on her checking account. "In case of emergency," she always said. She meant my emergency, not hers. Now, however, the emergency was hers, and the fact that her bank account was in both our names was helpful. I paid the bills, signing my own name to each check.

For the first time, I recognized that my mother had a serious mental problem.

She had acted strangely about resigning from her job. She had become unreasonably upset when she thought she would no longer be able to drive a car. She had stopped playing bridge. She had refused to look at apartments near her sisters after travelling over three thousand miles for that purpose. She had rejected the idea of moving into a retirement home, even though she had been considering such a move for several years. She had told people that her granddaughter would not do the grocery shopping, when the freezer and the shelves were loaded with food. She had refused to eat. She had said she was not receiving Social Security checks, though she had been getting them for ten years and they were still coming regularly.

None of these events had seemed serious to me; I had managed to find a reasonable explanation for each one. But when I sat beside her at that card table and she merely stared at her checkbook, repeating the same question over and over, I knew that something was wrong.

CHAPTER II

Some Definitions

When my mother was seventy she said to me, "The only thing that worries me about getting old is senility."

I did not take her seriously; in fact, I teased her about being redundant, for one meaning of senility is "characteristic of old age," and I told her that I did not see how one could become old without developing some of the characteristics of age: absent-mindedness, mild forgetfulness, physical weakness, for example. I was forty-nine at the time, usually more absent-minded and forgetful than she was, and probably no stronger physically. We come from a healthy, long-lived family. To cheer her up I reminded her of all this, and recalled the old joke about the man who said that he didn't mind getting older when he considered the alternative.

I do not know why I remember that conversation, which seemed unimportant at the time, but I have since wondered if she had some kind of premonition, or if even then she was aware of some symptoms which worried her. And I am still not certain what she meant by *senility*.

According to the AMERICAN HERITAGE DICTIONARY,[1] *senile* means *pertaining to, characteristic of, or proceeding from old age,* and *senility* means *the state of being senile.* A second definition for *senility*, however, *is mental and physical deterioration with old age.* This is the meaning most often given to the word today, as we begin to recognize the nature of diseases usually (but not always) related to old age.

The vagueness of the term *senility* is becoming apparent; it has been called a "wastebasket diagnosis" by at least two writers on aging.[2] It is not a true medical diagnosis, but a term for many symptoms, such as forgetfulness, loss of ability to concentrate, disorientation, lessening of emotional responses to others, and physical deterioration. These may be symptoms

17

of hardening of the brain arteries, destruction of the central nervous system, or chronic brain disease, all irreversible conditions. These same symptoms, however, may indicate anemia, vitamin deficiency, depression, or reaction to drugs, all of which can be cured or prevented. One doctor has suggested *emotional and mental disorders in old age* as a more accurate term than *senility*.

The phrase is more precise, but lengthy, awkward, and even misleading; for recently it has been discovered that some of the disorders that often affect older people can also occur in younger ones. Severe depression, for example, can occur in young children as well as in adults. *Mental disorders*, furthermore, can be easily confused with *mental illness*, and for some purposes these conditions are quite different. Examples of mental illness are schizophrenia, paranoia, and manic depression. Though the difference between a disorder and an illness is still not clear to me, I do know that financial aid is available for the latter, but not the former. (See Chapter VIII)

A shorter and more accurate term is *senile dementia*, or better yet, simply *dementia*, which is formed from Latin *de* (away from) and *mens* (mind), and defined in the AMERICAN HERITAGE DICTIONARY as "Irreversible deterioration of intellectual faculties with concomitant emotional disturbance resulting from organic brain disorder."

Senile dementia is defined as "progressive, abnormally accelerated deterioration of mental faculties and emotional stability in old age." *Presenile dementia* occurs in people younger than sixty or sixty-five, depending on whose book or article one is reading. According to a 1981 television broadcast, the actress Rita Hayworth has been suffering from presenile dementia; at the time of the broadcast she was sixty-one and had been institutionalized for many years because of her condition. One wonders: does presenile dementia become senile dementia when one reaches a certain age?

Miss Hayworth's condition has also been called *Alzheimer's disease*. Although this disease was described in 1906 by Alois Alzheimer, a German neurologist, little has been written about it until recently. It is characterized by a tangle of filaments and by groups of degenerated nerve endings, called *plaques*, in the cortex of the brain.

For the layman, the terminology continues to be confusing. A recent (1981) publication of the Johns Hopkins University School of Medicine states that Alzheimer's disease can be confirmed only by an autopsy.[3] If this is true, then how does one know that Miss Hayworth and others are victims of this disease? Recently a man in a Texas nursing home was shot by his brother because of the man's hopeless and incurable condition, diagnosed as Alzheimer's disease. How did the doctors know? To be fair, it must be stated that the diagnosis even without an autopsy was probably correct; such a diagnosis is made by the process of elimination.

Research in disorders of the brain is proceeding so rapidly that it is impossible to keep up with what is happening. It is possible, however, that the term *Alzheimer's disease* is sometimes used carelessly by journalists and even by doctors; it may become a euphemism for senility. A disease named for a person seems less offensive than one that describes a condition; Parkinson's disease, Huntington's chorea, even Hansen's disease come to mind. I must confess that I would have preferred telling people that my mother had Alzheimer's disease to saying that she was senile, and I am certain that she would have taken some comfort in having a disease with a name. Unfortunately I did not hear the term until after her death, having been too busy taking care of her to read up on mental disorders.

It is now becoming a household word, however. An NBC drama called "The Trouble with Grandpa" depicts the relationship between a seventeen-year-old girl and her grandfather, who is afraid of becoming senile. The girl consults a doctor about her grandfather's condition and is told that the old man may have Alzheimer's disease. The doctor suggests an examination, and one gets the impression that an office call will take care of it. The fact is that if the disease *can* be accurately diagnosed while the patient is still alive, it must be done with extremely sophisticated methods and newly-developed devices for scanning the brain.

In 1970 my mother's condition was diagnosed as *cerebral arteriosclerosis*, which is the narrowing of blood vessels in the brain, causing a reduction in the supply of oxygen. While Lawrence Galton refers to the "tendency to link senility with just one thing—hardening of brain arteries and chronic brain disease,"[4] Jane Otten and Florence D. Shelley distinguish between these two conditions:

> . . . arteriosclerosis . . . narrows the blood vessels in the brain and reduces the oxygen supply . . . this condition accounts for only a small fraction of the cases. Most of the senile are suffering from chronic brain disease, a destructive disease of the brain that robs them of their intellectual capacities, their emotional and physical control, their judgment, and their orientation to reality. Some physicians now refer to this as chronic brain disease (CBD), others as senile dementia. Some call it Alzheimer's disease, which is more properly identified with presenile dementia.[5]

One is tempted, at this point, to go back to the custom of covering all of the conditions mentioned so far (senile dementia, presenile dementia, cerebral arteriosclerosis, chronic brain disease, Alzheimer's disease) with that convenient wastebasket term, senility. And that isn't all: another condition thrown into this wastebasket is *atherosclerosis*, a particular kind of arteriosclerosis. A refreshingly clear distinction is made by Richard L. Landau, M.D. and Claire Landau:

> Strictly speaking, atherosclerosis refers to fatty deposits in the walls of the arteries, and arteriosclerosis to a more generalized development of arterial disease characterized by a loss of elasticity, hardening of the artery walls, and diminution of their caliber. In practice doctors often use the terms interchangeably because atherosclerotic lesions are the most important factor in the development of arteriosclerotic disease.[6]

The difficulty in keeping these terms straight is illustrated in Madeleine l'Engle's *The Summer of the Great-Grandmother:*

> I asked Pat, "What do you call it? Arteriosclerosis? Atherosclerosis?" "Most people say arterio, but it's athero."[7]

When Madeleine l'Engle's book was first published in 1974, a reviewer described its content as "an almost taboo subject of senility and old age." Recently this subject, fortunately, has been brought out of the closet; perhaps now the terms used to describe it will become more accurate. A few years ago a child who was afflicted by premature aging was described on television as *senile*. In 1981, three cases (two boys, aged eight and nine, and a woman of twenty-six) received considerable publicity but their condition was consistently and accurately called *progeria*, not senility. Progeria is a disease that ages its victims about ten times faster than is normal. It has nothing to do, apparently, with dementia. But it, too, has come out of the closet. The publicity given the two young boys is said to have changed their outlook on life and must have brightened the lives of other progeria victims and their parents.

Getting embarrassing conditions out into the open is the first step in doing something to help the victims. In the past, people with mental disorders or with physical deformities were kept out of sight by their families. There have been times in our history when those who behaved strangely were burned as witches. We are making some progress, though I realize that many nursing homes and mental institutions indicate by their conditions that the progress is slow. In fact, some people who look back to the time when families were larger, servants were more easily available, and the senile stayed at home, feel that we have gone backward rather than forward.

I was never embarrassed by my mother's condition, but it was evident that she was, and she was very clever at concealing it. When friends came to the house or when she met people at her church she would ask, quite charmingly, "And how is the family?" Probably she had no idea who the person was. But how resourceful of her to ask such an ambiguous question! Everybody has a family. She never said, "How are your children?" or "How is your mother?" or even, "How is *your* family?" but always "How is *the* family?" If a person had no family at all (not likely) he could interpret my mother's question to refer to the family with whom he lived, or even the family next door or perhaps a family of kittens!

Mother did not want me to talk about her condition with anyone, not even her minister. When I told her that I discussed with him her insistence that some of her furniture was being used by the church (it wasn't, of course), she was hurt. "If you had a problem with your mind," she said to me, "*I* wouldn't tell anybody about it."

On the other hand, at times she was quite candid. "I am *non compos mentis*," she might say to a person she had just met. And she often told me, when she was living at home with me, that she thought she should be in a hospital.

I wish now that I had talked frankly to her about her condition, perhaps early in the mornings, when she was least confused. But it is hard to say to someone, "There is something wrong with your mind," even though you both know that it is true.

It was also difficult for me to talk to doctors about her, but for different reasons. It was not easy to act as a go-between, and Mother was incapable of helping the doctor diagnose her problem herself. Furthermore, I felt guilty about taking up a doctor's time on what seemed an incurable and untreatable condition; and sometimes I suspected that the doctor did not understand the condition.

More important, the doctor did not really know my mother and I longed for the days of the "family doctor." When I was a child our doctor came to the house to treat my grandparents, my mother, my aunts, my cousins, and me. No doubt he knew less than doctors know today and he did not have access to the modern facilities, the drugs, and the treatments that are now available, but he knew *us.* I suspect that one reason various forms of dementia go undetected nowadays is that doctors no longer know their patients well. How can they, when they charge $35 for a five-minute visit?

I was told by several doctors that my mother's condition was "terminal." And what did that mean? Unable to elicit a satisfactory answer from any of her doctors, I called an elderly cousin who had retired from practicing medicine. I described Mother's condition and asked him how long she might be expected to live. I needed to know, for I was concerned not only about her physical and mental condition but also about her finances. Should I spend her money (on her, of course) with reckless abandon, assuming that she had only a few months to live? Or should I use it cautiously, perhaps supplementing her income with some of mine in order to stretch hers over several years?

My cousin answered without hesitation that my mother could live for another twenty years. I am still wondering why the other doctors referred to her condition as "terminal." She lived for over ten years, and she did not die of cerebral arteriosclerosis, that "terminal" disease, but of pneumonia. It is only fair to say that she probably contracted pneumonia, at the age of eighty-seven, partly as a result of inactivity, the result of her weakened physical condition, which in turn was a result of her limited mental capacity, which was caused by the arteriosclerosis. One could say that arteriosclerosis was an indirect and contributing cause of her death, but neither a direct nor an essential cause.

Why didn't the doctors refer to her condition as irreversible (which was true) rather than terminal? Perhaps medical students should be required to take a course in semantics.

With a relative who is seriously ill, especially one who is unable to communicate clearly, a doctor is needed who has time for her, who is aware of her emotional as well as her physical and mental problems, and who can give sympathetic advice to her family. Except on television soap operas and in comic strips such doctors are almost non-existent.

I was fortunate enough to have two such doctors for my mother, both of them assigned to the college where I was teaching. I deeply appreciate the personal interest they took in her. They did not dismiss her case as "terminal," but did what they could to make her comfortable and to help me care for her.

Before I put her under their care, her condition had been diagnosed twice: first as cerebral arteriosclerosis and later as "calcium deposits on the brain." So I still do not know whether she had arteriosclerosis or, possibly, chronic brain disease, or indeed whether or not there is any genuine difference between the two. By "calcium deposits" was the doctor who examined her referring to the plaques which indicated Alzheimer's disease? At the time, I had not heard of the disease. In either case, her condition was irreversible, and there was nothing that could be done for her except to try to keep her calm and comfortable and as contented as possible.

There are cases, however, in which patients who display the same symptoms that my mother had are *not* suffering from an irreversible disease. One such condition is depression. According to Otten and Shelley, the tendency is to neglect elderly people who are depressed, but it is possible to treat them successfully.[8] Symptoms include helplessness, hopelessness, loss of appetite, and loss of weight. The condition may start out as neurotic depression, caused by an external event such as the death of a husband or wife. It may then become psychotic, that is to say a condition caused by internal rather than external events. It may have an organic cause, such as hormonal abnormalities. Both physical and psychiatric treatment may thus be needed.

Elderly people sometimes consider depression a weakness and deny it, covering their condition by complaining of headaches, which they consider more respectable. Their symptoms are often similar to those of dementia. For example, they may be unable to answer simple questions; they may also become confused, forgetful, and disoriented.

Feelings of grief, guilt, depression, loneliness, despair, anxiety, or helplessness are not mental disorders, but if they remain unsolved and cause problems in functioning, outside help is needed. They may become mental illnesses or disorders. The point at which they become organic rather than functional is hard to distinguish. Organic disorders have a physical cause, while functional disorders are related to one's personality and experience.[9]

Organic disorders may be reversible or chronic. Chronic (that is, irreversible) disorders include the true dementias. Reversible disorders may be the result of malnutrition, anemia, adverse reactions to medication, tumors, or infection. I know from experience that medication can have strange and disturbing effects on a patient.

When Mother was in a hospital undergoing extensive tests, she was in a ward with five other people. I or another member of our family—one of her sisters or nieces or cousins—was by her side constantly, except for the few hours at night for which we hired a "sitter." When she was awake she fantasized constantly. She thought that the other people in the ward were there to play bridge, and that she was in charge. Her delusions were different from those she had under other circumstances (when she admittedly did not know where she was, for example, or when she thought that her furniture had been taken to the church), and I am certain that they were drug-induced. Several years later, when at my request her doctor prescribed a tranquilizer that I could give her at home, her reaction to it was severe depression, so I discontinued the medicine.

I sometimes wonder how many elderly people sent to a hospital with a physical problem, such as a broken hip, become disoriented or depressed because of the drugs they are given and are henceforth considered "senile" by their families.

When what appears to be dementia is discovered to be a reversible condition, the results are often dramatic. Lawrence Galton tells of sixty-six-year-old former judge, so confused and disoriented that he was believed to be "hopelessly senile," who was found to be suffering from hydrocephalus, or "water on the brain," a condition usually associated with children rather than older people. Two days after an operation to correct the hydrocephalus, the former judge was "alert, cheerful, oriented, functioning normally."[10]

Finally, there is a condition, irreversible but not serious, from which we all probably suffer to a certain extent, benign forgetfulness. We lose some of our neurons (brain cells) as we grow old, and we do not generate new ones. As a result of this loss we may become forgetful and less creative and take longer to process information. This condition should not be confused with dementia.

Neither should true dementia, of whatever form—arteriosclerosis, Alzheimer's disease, chronic brain damage—or other serious conditions, such as brain tumor, depression, or hydrocephalus, be dismissed as "only senility." Proper diagnosis is of utmost importance. If forgetfulness and occasional disorientation is nothing more than benign forgetfulness, the persons concerned can all rejoice and be happy. If the condition is reversible, appropriate steps can be taken. If it is not treatable, neither the person concerned nor his relatives need despair. Plans can be made, before the patient's condition gets worse, to make his last ten or twenty years as comfortable as possible under the circumstances.

Notes to Chapter II

1. ©1982 Houghton Mifflin Company. Reprinted by permission from *The American Heritage Dictionary of the English Language, second college edition.*

2. Lawrence Galton, Parade Magazine, June 29, 1975, p. 5. Robert N. Butler, *Why Survive? Being Old in America.* New York: Harper & Row, 1975, p. 232

3. Nancy L. Mace and Peter V. Rabins, M.D., *The 36-Hour Day.* Baltimore: The Johns Hopkins University Press, 1981, p. 88

4. Galton, p. 36

5. Jane Otten and Florence D. Shelley, *When Your Parents Grow Old.* New York: New American Library, 1976, p. 188

6. *50 Plus Magazine*, November 1981, p. 65

7. Madeleine l'Engle, *The Summer of the Great-Grandmother.* New York: Farrar, Straus and Giroux, 1974, p. 28

8. Otten and Shelley, pp. 192-94

9. Butler, p. 226

10. Galton, Parade Magazine, p. 5

CHAPTER III

The Patient At Home: What To Expect

When a relative for whom one is responsible becomes incapable of caring for herself, and when her case has been diagnosed as Alzheimer's disease, cerebral arteriosclerosis, or some other irreversible condition, what can be done for her? There are four possibilities.

She can be left in her own home with someone taking care of her.

If her family is large and not all family members in a household work or go to school, she can be moved into the home and the family can care for her.

If everyone in the family works or goes to school, she can still live with them but outside help will be needed as she cannot be left alone for long periods of time. The smaller the family the more outside help will be needed. When there is only one family member to care for the patient live-in help will probably be required.

Finally, if all else fails, she can be put in a nursing home or some other type of institution.

Leaving the patient in her own home with caretakers has advantages. She will probably be more contented than she would be anywhere else. The other family members can go on about their business, knowing she is being cared for and relieved that they have not put her in an institution.

While such an arrangement may seem ideal, some serious problems will undoubtedly arise. A reliable housekeeper must be found; and since there will be times when the housekeeper will have to go out shopping or to take care of her own needs—trips to a doctor or dentist, for example—someone else must be available to take her place. The ideal person for this job is a relative who is both needy and saintly and who has no other obligations. Few outsiders are willing to assume such a responsibility unless they are adequately paid, and adequate pay for such work means, as a rule, over a thousand dollars a month. I know of families who have paid two thousand and even that amount was not enough to keep the same person for any length of time.

Such a position requires the patience of Job and the fortitude of David. It means being not only manager of a house, but also cook, nurse, and companion. The housekeeping part includes managing money, shopping for groceries, preparing meals, seeing that the house is cleaned (probably someone else can be employed to clean it once a week or so), and taking care of emergencies involving heating, plumbing and electricity. The nursing duties include helping the patient get dressed and undressed, seeing that she eats balanced food, helping her find things that she loses, and keeping her as contented as possible.

If the patient or her relatives could afford to employ a separate housekeeper, cook, person to clean, nurse, and companion, the situation would be ideal. In other words, what is needed is the downstairs staff of the television series *Upstairs, Downstairs*. Obviously such an arrangement is not possible for most people. A more practical solution is to move the patient into the home of other family members. Even so there will be problems.

For one thing, there will probably be family disagreements. Since I am an only child, the primary responsibility for my mother was not shared; fortunately my extended family, consisting of countless cousins, three aunts, and an uncle by marriage, were helpful and supportive. Nevertheless, they did not always agree on what would be best for my mother.

Two of my aunts, both widows, lived together. One wanted Mother to move in with them, and from Mother's point of view that would have been quite satisfactory, I believe. But Mother's behavior was becoming more and more bizarre, and the other aunt said that if Mother moved in, she would move out. I do not believe that she was serious about leaving. Nevertheless, these two aunts had lived together for many years while Mother, by choice, had lived thousands of miles away from them. I could not let her condition cause a rift between them.

The other aunt, Mother's youngest sister, was keeping house for herself and her husband. She was willing to keep Mother until I could make other arrangements, but not indefinitely. "Put Sallie in a nursing home," she suggested, adding that there was an excellent one a few blocks from her house and that she would be glad to visit Mother often and to take care of her laundry and do whatever else was needed.

"I have always maintained," said the aunt who wanted Mother to live with her, "that no member of my family would ever go to one of those places. People are just put there to die."

We did put Mother in the nursing home, but after a few months I moved her to my house. I was then living several hundred miles from my aunts, and I knew that taking care of her while working at a full time job would be difficult. Essie, a woman who was helping with Mother at the nursing home, agreed to go home with us and to take care of Mother for me. Essie stayed with us less than a year; Mother lived in my home for five years, during which time we tried several different arrangements.

Essie stayed with us from October until April; she was more than satisfactory during that time. In addition to being efficient and industrious and showing almost infinite patience with my mother, she was an excellent cook. At first I did the cooking, thinking that Essie had enough to do to watch Mother twenty-four hours a day. But after Mother could do more for herself and required less attention, Essie began to prepare the meals. Although Mother's mental condition did not improve, she gained weight and seemed stronger physically.

No matter how good outside help is, however, there is a kind of disruption to one's life that accompanies having an outsider in the home. Essie herself needed some attention from me. She did not have a car, nor did she drive, and we were living in a small town with no public transportation. So when I gave her a day off every Thursday, I drove her to a larger town to do her shopping or any other errands that were necessary. This meant employing another woman to replace Essie on those days. I also took Essie to church on Sundays, a somewhat complicated procedure since she wanted to go to a church fourteen miles away from us.

When spring came, Essie decided to return to her home and plant her garden. I knew that she missed her home and her relatives, and I did not try to dissuade her from leaving.

I was paying her four hundred dollars a month, plus room and board, when she left in 1971. Her replacement, whom I procured by answering an advertisement, asked only three hundred, but she did not stay on week-ends. Ten years later I would have had to pay at least eight hundred a month for someone like Essie, and probably over a thousand.

Mrs. N., Essie's replacement, was something of a disaster. Like Essie, she shared a room with my mother. (I was in the process of adding two more rooms and another bathroom to the house, but they were not finished until shortly before my son and his family arrived.) The first day I showed her where Mother's nightclothes were and told her that although Mother could undress herself and put on her nightgown, she would need a little help and considerable supervision.

That evening I went to a friend's house for dinner and when I returned I looked into Mother's room, where I found Mother standing, fully clothed and completely bewildered, in the middle of the room. The new "helper" peeked out from under her covers and watched me help Mother get ready for bed. The next evening I again explained to her what assistance Mother would need, and Mrs. N. was somewhat more helpful.

Although Mother had to be constantly watched, there was relatively little to do for her. Essie had found that getting Mother dressed and undressed, helping her with her bath, seeing that she took her vitamins and medicine, and perhaps accompanying her on brief walks, still left plenty of time, so she had taken over the job of preparing the evening meal for all three of us. Mrs. N. had time on her hands but there seemed to be little that she was willing to do. Much of her time was spent on the telephone giving advice to members of her church who were having problems instead of paying attention to Mother's simple needs or keeping busy with light chores around the house. Mother had never felt neglected while Essie was fixing dinner; in fact, at times Essie found simple ways in which Mother could help. But she did resent Mrs. N's long telephone conversations, an activity from which she was completely excluded.

Obviously Mrs. N. was bored with the job. It was much more interesting to play Dear Abby than to take care of a mentally deranged woman. But I kept her until my son and his family arrived; she was a bridge between life with Essie and life with the family.

From Mother's point of view, the most satisfactory arrangement was having my son, his wife, and their children live with us. We were then a real family, four generations in fact. Living with the family as long as possible is usually recommended for anyone with dementia, and I know that Mother felt more secure with all of us around her than she did at any other time. For the rest of us, however, the situation was often troublesome and sometimes almost frightening.

My son had brought his wife and children from the west coast after Mother had been with me for almost a year, and they stayed with us several months before finding a place of their own. The children consisted of Michael, age three; Sarah, eighteen months; and David, an infant.

Mother adored David. When she sat in a rocker, we would put him in her arms, and she seemed delighted. But at times she would pick him up from a bed and walk around the house with him, even though we asked her not to. She was very careful, and probably the danger was minimal, but it still seemed a bit reckless to let her carry him. She could not remember that we had asked her not to walk with the baby.

Next to rocking and carrying David, she enjoyed chasing three-year-old Michael, usually when he had done something she considered naughty, but sometimes just for the sport of chasing him. If she thought he had been naughty, and she caught him, she would shake him. Michael sometimes deserved a shaking, but it seemed unfair to permit his mentally incompetent great-grandmother to discipline him.

The children survived all this, and for a while we four adults enjoyed being part of a big family. I bragged to our friends that we had established a new style of commune—a family of four generations. However, after about six months my daughter-in-law, a sensible young woman, found another house for herself, my son, and the children.

Why couldn't we manage longer? Mother seemed reasonably contented, though usually confused; I enjoyed having the children around; it was an economical way for all of us to live. But although the house was large enough for all of us, it had not been designed for children. It is all on one floor and has neither basement nor attic for play space. The floors are not carpeted; the living-room ceiling is high, and so is the noise level. It was hard to find a time or place to relax, partly because in the midst of all the hustle and bustle of the rest of the family, Mother demanded attention. She was especially concerned at this time about her money; I spent many hours going over her bank account with her, explaining where her money came from and what it was being spent for. Everything had to be repeated countless times. My son generously offered to answer her questions to relieve me of this time-consuming and fruitless chore, but Mother insisted that I do it.

When my son and his family left, Mother announced that she was able to stay at home alone while I went to work. We tried this for a while; she even prepared lunch for the two of us and had it ready when I came home at noon. Sometimes it was a strange lunch—once, for example, we had tuna salad which included maraschino cherries. I could have put up with the strange lunches, but being alone seemed, after a short time, to be making her regress. She was becoming more and more disoriented and confused, and we needed help.I then employed a nineteen-year-old married woman, who sometimes brought her baby along. Ina was to come for six or eight hours a day during the time I was at work. She was a shy young person and had a little trouble adjusting to my mother, who never seemed to realize that people were there to take care of her. She usually thought that she was taking care of them.

"Well," Mother said to me after Ina's first day with her, "I have been baby-sitting all day." She meant with Ina herself, who had not brought the baby that time!

After a week or so, however, Mother and Ina got along fine, especially when Ina brought her baby with her. Usually she left it with a cousin, but we found that the baby entertained Mother. Since Ina had little to do except stay with

Mother, help her take a bath, and give her lunch, she could watch both Mother and the child almost constantly. Ina's baby was almost a year old and rather heavy for his age, so Mother was not tempted to pick him up as she had picked up little David.

The only problem was that Ina had to leave about four every afternoon, when her husband was free to come for her. He was a patient young man and never complained if he had to wait, sometimes as much as an hour, until I got home from work. I felt pressured, however, as it did not seem fair to keep Ina, her husband, and the baby waiting so long. Mother could have been left alone for a short time each afternoon, but Ina was too conscientious to leave until I returned from work.

Ina quit working for us when she was going to have another baby, and for a while my daughter-in-law's sister, who had moved to our town, took care of Mother. She was an artist, and thinking that Mother might be entertained by watching her work, I suggested that she bring her easel and paints to the house. Mother always liked to see people working; in fact, next to working herself, I believe it was what made her happiest. But apparently Mother did not consider painting landscapes legitimate work. Fortunately, a few months after Ina's baby was born Ina was able to leave both her children with a cousin and return to stay with Mother during the day.

In the five years that Mother stayed with me, I employed not only Essie, Mrs. N., Ina, my daughter-in-law's sister, and a woman to take care of Mother on Essie's day off and at other times when I needed someone in an emergency; I also employed another woman to take care of Mother for two weeks while I went to Mexico for a much-needed vacation. In some ways she was quite satisfactory, but she talked to me in front of Mother as if Mother were not present. Even though Mother was not mentally alert, she remained sensitive to her surroundings. I was concerned about leaving her alone with this thoughtless woman; however, when I returned from Mexico all was well.

Finding and keeping a good caretaker for a person with dementia is not easy, but doing without one is impossible. To cope with dementia in one's home, some kind of outside help is essential. And to make the situation bearable, one needs also good friends and supportive relatives. I was fortunate in having both.

One of Mother's sisters had gone, together with her husband, to get Mother and bring her back to her home until I could make other arrangements. Another sister had offered to take her into her home, an offer which was not accepted but which nevertheless I appreciated. A cousin had taken care of Mother for a few days to relieve my aunt and her husband of some of the strain. All of this was particularly helpful, and since Mother had visited all these members of the family often, she was not a stranger in their homes. Ordinarily, moving a person in Mother's condition from house to house would be inadvisable, but Mother seemed cheered somewhat by all the attention she was getting. When I put her in a nursing home near them, her relatives visited her often, especially after I had to leave to begin my school year. By the time I left, I had decided to return for her and move her to my house as soon as I could get it ready.

The question was how to get her there, as the plane trip involved changing in Atlanta, a wait-over there of several hours, and then a forty-mile drive once we reached the airport nearest my house. It could have been done; after all, my aunt and uncle had moved her four or five times that far. And since Essie had agreed to travel with us, we surely could have managed, though I was not looking forward to the trip.

As it turned out, we flew in a private plane owned by the husband of one of my cousins. Moving my mother in this fashion was an act of generosity which I shall never forget. Five of us—the plane's owner, the pilot, Mother, Essie, and I—took the trip together in less than half the time it would have taken by commercial plane, and in greater comfort.

Friends, as well as relatives, can be a tremendous help in times of crisis—and living with a dementia patient can appear to be a continuing crisis. I was especially fortunate in both our relatives and our friends. Those friends who lived in town came to see us often, always treating Mother with respect and courtesy, never expressing surprise at her behavior no matter how bizarre it might be. For her part Mother, who had always enjoyed parties, behaved better when we had guests than when we were alone.

The major problem I had when I had invited people to dinner was in controlling Mother before they came. She wanted to help. I would let her set the table, but then I had to re-set it while she wasn't looking, as she was as likely as not to give all the knives to one guest and all the spoons to another.

A bachelor friend of ours, who had often visited us on his way to see his relatives in a nearby state, generously offered to stay with Mother for three weeks so that I could go to Europe. A relentless traveler himself, he persuaded me that I both needed and deserved such a trip. I shall be forever grateful for his generosity in taking care of my mother.

At the time, Mother was in good physical condition and could take her bath unaided, though someone needed to fill the tub with water for her. The tub was equipped with handles so that she could get herself in and out of it alone.

Our friend George is a gourmet cook, so I am sure that Mother had better meals than she had ever had before in her life, with the possible exception of those that Essie prepared. He also showed great patience in dealing with her mental aberrations. It took tremendous patience to deal with her as it does with all people in her condition. When I would come home from work, for example, we had a kind of ritual conversation almost every day.

"Tell me," she would begin, as if we were strangers, "What are the children's names?"

"Michael, Sarah, David, and Jeremiah," I would reply. By this time Michael was six, Sarah was four, David was three, and Jeremiah, who had been born after my son's family moved to their own house, was a year old.

After a pause of about thirty seconds Mother would repeat the question and I would repeat the answer. The same conversation could last for thirty minutes or longer. When I returned from Europe, George reported that he and Mother had had this same lengthy and repetitive conversation every day that I had been gone.

Short-term forgetfulness is one universal characteristic of dementia. Confusion is another. Sometimes Mother could not remember who I was. At times, when we were having one of these repetitious conversations, she would introduce a variation. "Tell me," she would ask, "What relation are you to me?" The first time she asked me this question I had to try hard to conceal my surprise that she did not know.

"I'm your daughter," I would reply, and she seemed quite satisfied with the answer, never indicating that there was anything unusual in her not knowing me.

She remembered that she had a daughter named Dorothy, but quite often she did not recognize me as that daughter. One night she got out of her bed, came to my room, and asked pathetically, "What ever happened to Dorothy?" When I assured her that I was Dorothy, she seemed satisfied and went back to bed. Though such behavior as this is pathetic indeed, it is comforting to know that a person in Mother's condition can often be reassured easily. What such a person needs more often than anything else, I believe, is reassurance.

A friend of mine sometimes stayed with Mother when I had to go to an evening faculty meeting. On one of these occasions, as I was walking down the driveway to get in my car, Mother looked out the window and said to my friend, "Who is that woman?" My friend told me later that that was her first recognition of the seriousnes of my mother's condition.

In addition to loss of short-term memory and failure to recognize people, dementia patients suffer from disorientation. They do not know where they are. I have heard of people who have lived in the same house for over thirty years, who insisted constantly that they wanted to *go home*. Occasionally, Mother expressed a desire to go home, but as a rule she asked to go to "the other house."

I would sometimes drive her around town, asking her to direct me to the house she meant, hoping to convince her that there was no other house that we owned or rented. This was an exercise in futility. She enjoyed the ride but when we returned home she would say, "Shouldn't we go to the other house now?" or sometimes, "I didn't shut the windows in the other house. We'd better go see about them."

There were times when she did not recognize our house as a home but thought it was a church or a railroad station.

"What are all my things doing here?" she would ask in alarm.

Although Mother's brain was obviously diseased, there were some parts of it which were functioning as well as mine, perhaps better. One was her long-term memory. As a child, she had lived in a town about fifty miles south of where we lived when she came to stay with me. She had not been there for over sixty years but she remembered the name of the main street, Saloon Street. Once we drove there to locate this street, which she described as having, as one would expect of a street by that name, numerous saloons. When we arrived we learned that there was no longer a Saloon Street; but we were told that the street now called Main Street used to be Saloon Street back in pre-Prohibition days.

It was unwise to try to reason with my mother, but she could sometimes exhibit a strong ability to do her own reasoning. She was often able to conceal her disability from others, especially from people who did not know her very well. Her device of asking a person "How is the family?" was definitely an indication that part of her brain was still normal.

One of my biggest problems was Mother's possessiveness; she disliked my paying attention to anyone else. One summer my friend Frances, with whom I enjoy playing Scrabble, came to spend a few days with us. We never got out the Scrabble board until after Mother had gone to bed, and during the day we each gave her as much attention as we possibly could. But Mother would not stay in bed, nor would she join us at the Scrabble table. Instead, she persisted in wandering out to the living room and announcing that she did not know where she was supposed to sleep. Each time, I would lead her back to the bedroom.

With all those interruptions I lost every game. Finally I suggested to my friend that she take Mother to her room, and she agreed. The next time Mother interrupted us, I said, "It's my turn to play. Frances will show you where your bed is. Do you mind, Frances?"

"Of course not," Frances replied graciously, "I'll be glad to. Shall we go to your room now, Sallie?"

Mother drew herself up as tall as she could, adding, it seemed, another inch to her five-feet-two. "I should say not!"

she declared fiercely, turning on her heels and walking straight to her bedroom.

What did this behavior mean? Was she trying to make me pay attention to her? Or was she really confused and disoriented? If so, why did her behavior change so rapidly? Was she suddenly embarrassed into lucidity when she realized that our guest was going to take charge of her?

The truth is, I believe, that along with forgetfulness, confusion, and disorientation, there is sometimes a kind of self-centeredness which increases the longer one suffers from dementia—at least up until the extremely advanced stage, when the patient has lost the ability to relate to anyone, at any time, in any way. One needs to understand this self-centeredness and, as far as possible, accept it.

Two other characteristics sometimes manifest themselves in dementia patients: a tendency to wander and a tendency to violence. Fortunately, my mother never displayed either of these. Once she threatened to hit me with her walking stick, but I quietly left the room and she calmed down before I returned five minutes later. Since she had always been cautious, I did not worry about her wandering away from home, though one time she wrapped a few small possessions up in a shower cap, and a visiting friend, thinking that Mother was going to leave the house, persuaded her to sit down with the rest of us. I was busy talking to other guests, but noticed what was going on, and was waiting to see if Mother would really go outside. In that case I was prepared to go after her and bring her back. I have known of other dementia patients who often wandered, not only away from their home but from nursing homes as well.

Every case is different, just as every individual is different. What is surprising, however, are the similarities: the disorientation, the loss of short-term memory, the retention of long-term memory, the growing tendency to self-centeredness, and the bizarre behavior. In spite of a certain amount of predictability, one never knows what people with dementia will do next. Life with them is full of surprises, usually unpleasant ones; but if such situations are handled with care, the surprises are less likely to turn into disasters.

CHAPTER IV

The Patient At Home:
Some Practical Suggestions

Two years after the death of my mother, a friend began to observe the symptoms of senile dementia in hers. "I knew about the problem with your mother," she said to me, "but I did not really understand until the same thing occurred to mine."

Fortunately, there are now support groups for relatives of people with senile dementia. These groups have united to form a national organization, called the Alzheimer's Disease and Related Disorders Association (ADRDA), with headquarters in New York City. In 1981 there were twenty-five chapters,[1] and more have been formed since then. Such groups sponsor lectures by authorities who can offer help and guidance to families of dementia patients and, perhaps more important, give members an opportunity to exchange ideas.

Although such a group was not available to me while my mother was alive, I found it helpful to talk, whenever I could, with people who had parents or other relatives who exhibited some of my mother's symptoms. I was surprised to find that there were so many of us. I would have welcomed an opportunity to meet even more, and to have had the guidance that an organization such as ADRDA can give.

Most of the adjustments that I made at the time I cared for my mother were experimental. Some things worked; some did not. What worked for my mother and me will not necessarily work for other families, and what did not work for us may possibly work for someone else. There are many things which, if I had the opportunity, I would do differently.

When I started taking care of Mother, one of the first things I noticed was that she had trouble getting in and out of her dresses. That was a problem easily solved: I bought her dresses that buttoned down the front so that she could slip them on without having to lift her arms over her head. Even so, at first there was a little trouble helping her into them, as she seemed to have some stiffness in her arms and shoulders. We had to put them on her slowly and carefully.

Mother enjoyed shopping and I enjoyed buying clothes for her. She wore a size ten at first, but after gaining a little weight got up to a size twelve. Knowing her size, I could bring clothes home for her, as trying dresses on in a small dressing room would have been rather difficult for her. It is important to keep a patient looking nice, and I believe that I succeeded in this, with some help from her. She went shopping with me from time to time to select material and a pattern, and we had some dresses made for her by a patient and understanding dress-maker, who was even willing to come to our house occasionally and bring us pattern books. Mother, who had at one time sewed beautifully, was still knowledgeable about clothes.

She had always loved pretty clothes and was equally fond of attractive home furnishings. After I had our house enlarged we needed more bedroom furniture and I let Mother select some to be used in her room. After looking at a number of stores, she finally found a set of unusual and suitable chests and a mirror, which I still consider some of the prettiest bedroom furniture I have ever seen.

Mother has always been a tireless shopper and I do not like shopping at all, but I was happy to take her to look for clothes or furniture, as shopping was one thing that still gave meaning to her life. This kind of activity would not be suitable for everyone—certainly not for most men, and not for all women.

There were some things, however, that I thought Mother could still do, which she was not able to manage at all. At her own home she used to spend an hour or more a day, whenever it did not rain, watering the shrubbery and flowers. So once I arranged the hose for her, with the sprinkler attachment just right, and handed it to her. I even pointed it for her in the direction of the shrubs. She absent-mindedly turned the hose on the gravel walk and even with more assistance from me seemed unable to point it toward the plants she was supposed to be watering. Since she showed no interest in this activity I did not pursue it further.

She was good at shelling lima beans, however, and doing that made her feel useful, I believe. When I discovered that Mrs. N., the second helper I employed, could not cook and did not like house cleaning, I questioned her about what she liked to do and found that she enjoyed gardening. I have a large lot, and Mrs. N. showed me the best place for what she considered a small garden; to my city-bred eyes it seemed to be a small farm. We planted corn, beans, tomatoes, lettuce, and cucumbers. Mother was of no help in the garden—I had not expected her to be, but I thought she might like to watch Mrs. N. and me work in it. Unfortunately, when she went to the garden with us she would step on the plants, not seeming to recognize the difference between paths and rows. But she and Mrs. N. would sit on the back porch and shell our home-grown beans happily for an hour or so every morning during the season.

Incidentally, I developed a lasting interest in gardening. I still plant a garden every spring, on the same spot that Mrs. N. selected. It is a therapeutic hobby for anyone, and I believe that it would be especially good for a dementia patient, man or woman, who has gardened in the past.

Mother, I am sure, had shelled beans as a child, and was able to recall the simple movements needed for that activity. It has occurred to me that the ability of a patient to participate in an activity is related to the difference between long-term and short-term memory. It is generally believed that a dementia patient cannot learn anything new; nor can she, as anyone who has been around such patients knows, remember how to do everything that she has done in the past. (Mother could not remember how to water the plants, though she had done so before.) A knowledge of the patient's past activities is extremely helpful in taking care of her; that is, perhaps, the greatest advantage in keeping her at home as long as possible.

In the winter I tried to get Mother to knit, which she had been able to do at one time. My aunts and I attempted to interest her in knitting some squares for an afghan, but she was uncooperative. My daughter-in-law, several months later, was a little more successful at interesting Mother in this activity, and observed that Mother was fairly skillful at it. After a few minutes, however, Mother would put the needles and the yarn in her lap and stare into space. It may be that her hands were stiff.

Although this project was unsuccessful with my mother, knitting or crocheting might be a suitable activity for some patients, as long as the project is kept simple and the patient already knows how to do it.

Mother liked to be useful around the house. She was able to wash dishes, after I put the food away and got the water ready. We had a dishwasher, but as doing the dishes was good for her I seldom used it. Yet there were times when she would simply walk away from the kitchen, saying that she would wash the dishes later, which she never remembered to do.

Her favorite chore was sweeping the patio, and she did this thoroughly and well. The woman who came to clean house for us once a week told me that Mother would not let her sweep the patio, saying proudly, "That's my job." Sweeping is probably a therapeutic activity for anyone, male or female. I believe that people in nursing homes might be happier if allowed (but not required) to sweep their own rooms. Mother got the patio clean, but what is much more important, she enjoyed the activity and felt useful.

Several times I gave her a dust rag and asked her to dust the furniture, thinking that dusting was a simple activity which she could manage and which might give her pleasure. The trouble was she never moved from one piece of furniture to another, but stood wiping off the same piece over and over. Then she would put down the rag and wander away.

The best home therapy for Mother was work, whenever I could find something that she could do. I also tried to the best of my ability to keep her entertained. She enjoyed reading the newspaper, especially the ads. We subscribed to a daily paper published in the nearest big city, over a hundred miles away from us, and I could not make Mother understand that we weren't able to go to every sale advertised in the paper. I know now that I should not have tried to explain. I should simply have said, "Maybe we can go tomorrow."

The newspaper kept Mother oriented somewhat in time, if

not in space. She always looked at the date. I have read that it is a good idea to keep clocks and calendars in evidence, but I found the paper more useful. It became hard for her to tell time, and she paid little attention to calendars (after all, what good is a calendar if you know neither the day of the week or the date?), but she read the paper regularly every morning, always beginning with the date.

We had a black and white television set, which Mother never watched; in fact, she did not even like me to watch it. When I turned it on she would say, "How much longer are you going to be doing that?" or "When will that program be over?" Finally, with her appreciation of color in mind, I bought a color set, which she began to watch with me. Knowing that at one time she had enjoyed soap operas, I began watching *Search for Tomorrow* with her, and she seemed interested. I doubt that she followed the plot, but I believe that at times she was caught up in the emotions of the characters. Like many people, I'm a bit of a snob about soap operas, considering them a waste of time. Taking care of Mother gave me a chance to watch one without being haunted by the feeling that I should be doing something better with my time. Perhaps rationalizing, I told myself that Mother would not like to watch the TV alone.

Taking care of a dementia patient has its few small blessings.

In addition to this soap opera, we also watched *To Tell the Truth;* I shall always be grateful to Peggy Cass and Kitty Carlisle, two regulars on that program, for entertaining both of us. Miss Carlisle's elegant clothes were especially appealing to Mother.

Ordinarily Mother did not care much for the news, but she would watch it if I turned it on. She enjoyed certain newscasters, especially Irving R. Levine, whose precise and articulate speech pleased her.

Most of all, however, she enjoyed the Watergate trials—not because of what had happened, which she did not understand, but because of Pat Nixon who, she said, was one of her closest friends. According to Mother, Mrs. Nixon had on numerous occasions visited the high school where she taught, had spoken to the students often at assemblies, and had become a close friend of Mother's. It is true that President and Mrs. Nixon had once been in a parade that passed the high school. It is possible that Mrs. Nixon had visited the school, and she may have spoken at an assembly once. It is certain, however, that she and my mother had not been close friends; I would certainly have known it if they had been! But Mother's fantasized friendship with the first lady was harmless and I saw no reason to discourage it.

Most of the material which I have read has advised against encouraging fantasy, and has stressed "reality orientation." It seems to me that one should do whatever is expedient at the time. If believing that Pat Nixon was her friend made television programs more interesting to Mother, I saw no reason to argue with her about it.

I know a ninety-year-old woman in a nursing home who often writes letters to her mother and gives them to her niece to mail. The niece takes them quietly and destroys them later. That seems a reasonable thing to do. Why upset an old woman by arguing?

On the other hand, when my mother mentioned, as she sometimes did, that she wanted to go see her mother, I reminded her that her mother had been dead for over twenty years. Such reminders never seemed to upset her; if they had, I would have tried to think of some other response. The important thing is to keep the patient calm, whether by gently bringing her back to reality or by going along with her fantasy.

An interesting difference between insanity and senile dementia is the nature of fantasies. An insane person might imagine that she is living in a different century or that she is a historical character. The fantasies of a dementia patient are more reasonable and consequently often impossible for a stranger to recognize as mere fantasy. The patient may, for example, think herself in a different city or that her parents are still alive, but she would never believe herself to be on another planet or to be Marie Antoinette.

There is a middle road between insistence on reality and complete acquiescence to the patient's fantasy. Our friend

George was unusually resourceful in finding reasonable answers to Mother's unreasonable questions. Much of the furniture in our house was Mother's, and when she did not know where she was she would express concern about it. "What are all my lovely things doing here?" she would ask, thinking our house was a church or, sometimes, a railroad station. I tried to enlighten her, but with little success. George, when he stayed with her, would say simply, "I don't know, Sallie, but isn't it wonderful that they are here where we can enjoy them?" She sometimes looked a little puzzled at his answer, but it seemed to satisfy her.

There were a few occasions when I could reason with her by presenting concrete evidence. One day she insisted that my piano was hers. It is a small baby grand, standing in the middle of the living room with a couch behind it. Mother was sitting on the couch, and to make her point more emphatic she would bang on the top of the piano with her hand. I was afraid that she would hurt herself or even the piano, so I produced the receipt and the cancelled check with which I had paid for it. I did not expect her to capitulate. Like other attempts to calm her it was a shot in the dark, and I was surprised when it worked. She looked at the receipt, said "You're right," and dropped the subject.

Mother was aware of her mental problems, and during her lucid moments she would sometimes attempt to explain some of her strange behavior. Once she told me that the reason she became confused in the house, she thought, was because sometimes we entered through the front door and sometimes through the garage. With a little effort I could always take her through the same entrance, and after she pointed the problem out to me I did so. She still became disoriented, especially at night, but I believe that she was less frequently confused in the daytime.

I have talked with people who could calm a patient who was disoriented at home and who wanted to go "home" or "to the other house" by taking her for a ride. With Mother that did not work. When we returned she was always as confused as ever and immediately started asking to go to the other house.

She did enjoy going to church on Sundays, It was a chance

for her to dress up, to see people, and to listen to a sermon, which, she usually reported to me afterwards, was "simply out of this world." The music was soothing to her, also, I believe.

I tried playing soft music at home—Viennese waltzes, for example—on the stereo, but she did not particularly enjoy it. Perhaps she thought it was distracting me, that I was listening to it instead of to her. But I am sure that many people in her condition would be helped by music.

Pets have been found helpful in many cases. Essie had a dog, a part Collie named Tammy. Mother and Tammy paid no attention to each other; you might say that they lived in amiable unawareness of each other's presence. But many people in her condition would no doubt be helped by the presence of a pet.

Anyone taking care of a dementia patient needs occasional relief, and I was fortunate in being able to send Mother to visit her sisters from time to time. She was watched carefully all the way there and back, by relatives who put her on and took her off the plane and stewardesses who were instructed to take special care of her while she was aboard. Most books and articles advise against a change of residence for anyone in her condition, but she enjoyed the trips. After all, she was not going to be among strangers or even in houses where she had not stayed before.

Her sisters' health began to fail, however, and the visits had to be discontinued. It became harder for our relatives to make the trip to see her, also. Friends could not visit us all the time. Even though we were willing and able to pay for outside helpers, they were not always available. I kept her at home as long as I could, not wanting to put her in a nursing home. But taking care of her consumed, as the title of a useful handbook on taking care of dementia patients at home indicates, a "36-hour day."[2]

When a friend pointed out that the sacrifices I was making were out of all proportion to any good being done for my mother, I had to agree. And when Mother kept saying, as she often did, "I need more people around me," I decided that it was time to start looking for a place where she would have them. By this time she seldom knew who I was. It seemed pointless to keep her at home any longer.

Notes to Chapter IV

1. Linda Hubbard Getze, "They're Coping with 'Senility.'" *Modern Maturity,* April-May 1981, p. 82

2. Nancy L. Mace and Peter V. Rabins, M.D., *The 36-Hour Day: A Family Guide to Caring for Persons with Alzheimer's Disease, Related Dementing Illnesses, and Memory Loss in Later Life.* Baltimore: The Johns Hopkins University Press, 1981

CHAPTER V

Nursing Homes: What To Look For

As I look back on the five years when I kept my mother at home, I wonder how either of us survived the frustrations. There were times when Mother was happy, if only momentarily. She would sometimes look out the sliding glass doors at the rose bushes or the pine trees and say contentedly, "I am so blessed!" But such occasions were rare. More often she would say, "When are you going to take me home?" Or, "Couldn't I take that bus that goes by here every morning?" It was useless to keep informing her that the yellow bus was for school children only.

When I brought her to live with me I fully intended to keep her until she died; I even enlarged the house to provide a room for persons I would employ to stay with us and care for her. Enlarging the house was easy. Getting someone to stay, especially at a price we could afford, seemed impossible.

Keeping Mother contented was an even greater problem than obtaining helpers for her. She seemed especially unsuited to the quiet, semi-rural life we led. She enjoyed people and would have been less unhappy, I believe, if we could always have had guests.

By this time I was not a stranger to nursing homes. Mother had stayed temporarily in a comfortable and pleasant one in the city where her sisters lived and I had visited others. In spite of the horror stories about some of them, many are well-run and the patients are treated with respect and kindness. But even the best are not as pleasant for the patient as a real home, with her family. However, only a saint can provide a dementia patient with the constant attention she demands. Since few of us are saints, we have to settle for less: an institution, frequent visits, and the guilt feelings that go with such an arrangement. In such a place a patient gets less attention than at home, but she receives constant care and she is safe.

There are basically three types of facilities; many homes contain all three. They are Skilled Nursing Facilities (SNF), Intermediate Care Facilities (ICF), and Residential Care Facilities (RCF). A single institution may include only one type, all three types, or two types. There are also homes run by individual families, called Family Care Homes, which according to state regulations can care for a limited number of patients.

A Skilled Nursing Facility is needed if the patient has a serious chronic illness, is bedridden, or is convalescing from a stay in a hospital. In an SNF, twenty-four hour nursing service is provided. People with chronic brain disorders, such as my mother, are considered to have a chronic condition, not a chronic illness. They qualify for SNF only if they become ill with some other disease.

In an Intermediate Care Facility the patient will receive intermittent nursing service as needed. A licensed practical nurse is on duty at least most if not all of the time, and usually a registered nurse is in charge. Most patients in this kind of facility can feed themselves, can dress themselves with a little help, and are ambulatory or able to sit in a wheel chair for a good part of the day. In such facilities about half the patients have some form of dementia and are consequently disoriented and confused.

A Residential Care Facility is a non-medical institution in which patients are provided with minimal care. They may need occasional help with bathing and dressing and reminders to take medication, but they are lucid and able to be fairly self-sufficient.

The majority of people who enter a nursing home because of mental disorders need the Intermediate Care Facility, though they may be moved later to the SNF if needed, and in rare cases perhaps be moved to an RCF. I saw that happen to one charming elderly lady and heard her exclaim gleefully, "I've been promoted!"

Finding a suitable nursing home which has space available is not easy, and it is advisable to visit a number of homes before making a decision. This is not a pleasant chore; to the uninitiated even fairly good nursing homes are depressing places, and one's first reaction is to forget the whole idea and continue keeping the patient at home, regardless of almost unbearable frustrations. One sometimes finds, however, that first impressions are misleading, and that patients who seem pathetic are actually having everything possible done to keep them comfortable. Even an excellent staff cannot turn a nursing home into a resort hotel.

Naturally one wants the best possible care for the patient in the most pleasant surroundings possible. I believe that the three most important qualities to look for in a nursing home for a person with dementia are the cleanliness and attractiveness of the surroundings, the helpfulness of the staff, and the relative responsiveness of the patients—not necessarily in that order.

In most homes, not many patients are responsive to others, but a few are usually able to talk coherently and intelligently. Those who cannot talk, perhaps because of stroke, can often smile and respond to a touch on the shoulder. In 1970, before bringing my mother to live with me, I visited several homes just in case we would need one, and in one I was favorably impressed by the attitude of the patients, especially three neatly-dressed women in wheelchairs who spoke cheerfully to me, making favorable comments about the place and urging me to come back bringing my mother.

Unfortunately, when I took Mother there five years later to see if it would still be a good place for her, it had changed. The three cheerful ladies in wheelchairs were no longer there; perhaps they had gone home, or to some other nursing home. In fact, I saw no well-dressed and cheerful people at all; instead, I saw rows of patients in a long hallway, all in drab hospital gowns, staring blankly into space. The facility was three or four times as large as it had been five years earlier, it had changed management, and it had become a warehouse for old people, rather than a comfortable and pleasant place for them to live.

I was appalled, but Mother did not seem to notice the patients lined up against the wall. We went into a reception room and sat down in comfortable chairs, and she said, "This seems like a very nice place." It was indeed an attractive room, but I am sure that the patients spent little if any time there. Either Mother had not noticed their condition or she had forgotten what we had just seen. Her memory span usually was about thirty seconds. It is possible that she thought we planned to buy the building and that we would live in it by ourselves.

It has been suggested by some doctors that the patient be allowed to participate in selecting a home, but obviously that is not always possible. If my mother had been capable of selecting a nursing home, I would not have been putting her into one.

It may be that the patients had been put out in the hallway while their rooms were being cleaned. though why all rooms would have to be cleaned at the same time, with all occupants moved out as if they were furniture, is not clear to me. I was not so much disturbed by their being lined up (though it did not seem like an arrangement conducive to sociability) as by the blank expressions on their faces. I suspected that they had all been heavily sedated. The only good thing I noticed about this nursing home was that it was clean.

Absolute cleanliness is not always possible in these institutions, as there is bound to be a certain amount of incontinence, and one cannot expect the staff to be constantly standing by with a mop. If, however, the smell of urine is strong and always present, something is wrong. More important than the condition of the floors is the condition of the patients. Are they left unattended, with wet or soiled clothing? Are there adequate toilet facilities, and are the patients helped to use them at frequent enough intervals? If a bedridden patient is mentally capable of using his bell or light to summon an attendant when he needs a bedpan how quickly does one come?

Most institutions permit, even encourage patients to wear their own clothes; some do the patient's personal laundry, usually for an added fee. In some institutions a member of the family must take the patient's clothes home and wash them, an arrangement not too inconvenient for most families. In other institutions the patients wear hospital garments. Needless to say, these give a depressing air to the place, even though they are kept clean.

From my point of view, the most important thing to look for in an institution is the attitude of the staff, from the administrator to the floor-moppers. In fact, I would include, in addition to the staff, the family members who come to visit the patients.

My mother was in three institutions over a period of ten years. The first, near her sisters, was a one-story building arranged around a courtyard, where the patients could be taken out in their wheelchairs in good weather to enjoy the flowers and the grass. The manager and other members of the staff were all courteous and seemed to take a personal interest in the patients who looked well cared for. Mother shared a room with a family friend who was recuperating from a hip injury. Never having been in a hospital in her life, Mother did not understand the call bell system. When she wanted something, she would ask Thelma her roommate, who would then ring her bell and an attendant would come. Thelma was very gracious about all this, but when Mother began waking her several times during the night, the head nurse moved Thelma to another room where she could get some much-needed rest. Mother was then without a roommate for a while and no doubt she felt very lonely.

I went to see Mother almost daily, and at least one other member of our family went to see her every day, also. At first we thought that she could stay there indefinitely, but she did not like the idea at all. When visitors would remark about what a pleasant place it was and how fortunate she was to be living there, she would reply, "I do *not* live here," adding sometimes, if the visitor was a member of our family, "When can I go home?"

Eventually, however, she became better adjusted. After I left to begin my fall classes and to get my house ready for Mother, she expressed some doubt to her sisters about the advisability of leaving. "I am getting along so well here," she said once, adding, "What do you think I should do?"

"If I had a daughter who wanted me to come and live with her," one sister replied, "I would certainly go." Although over seventy, this sister of Mother's was still working every weekday in a government office, and she went every evening to see

Mother at the nursing home, which was across town from her home. Since I had not consented to letting Mother stay with her, she was determined to visit as frequently as possible, even though I am sure that these visits were physically and emotionally tiring. It was for her sake as much as for my mother's that I moved Mother to my house.

I thought when I moved her that there was a possibility I would have to put her in another nursing home, especially if her physical condition became worse. After she had lived with me for a few weeks, however, her appetite improved markedly; she ate everything that Essie cooked. She looked better, partly as a result of gaining weight and partly because I took her to the beauty parlor once a week to get her hair done. Also, Essie and I dressed her in becoming clothes. With improvements in her appearance came considerable improvement in morale.

If I could have kept Essie, or someone like her, I might have been able to keep Mother at home longer. When Essie was with us I could finish my school work at the office and when I came home I could give Mother my undivided attention, which she demanded. But when I had to rush home from school so that our helper could leave, or when the helper was so inefficient that I felt obligated to return early to prepare supper and to see that Mother was all right, the strain began to wear on me.

Most important, though Mother was in good physical health, her mental condition had not improved at all. In fact, it seemed to be growing steadily worse. There had been a time when she was lucid in the early mornings, but those periods of lucidity were becoming less and less frequent.

We lived only a few blocks from a hospital which had added an Extended Care Unit where patients could stay after an operation or treatment. Although it was part of a hospital, not a real nursing home, it had some of the characteristics of a nursing home: a lounge where the patients could gather to eat or watch television, an activity program for the patients, and parties on occasions such as Christmas and birthdays.

The major advantage was that it was near enough so that I could visit Mother frequently. Even more important, most of the other patients were visited often by their families. These visitors talked to my mother, and whenever possible I tried, in turn, to do small favors for the other patients.

For a year or so Mother shared a room with a woman whose sister, Mrs. W., came every day to eat lunch with her. At this time neither Mother nor her roommate seemed to want to go to the lounge for meals, but preferred sitting in their wheelchairs in their room. Mrs. W. brought her own lunch, which often contained delicacies that her sister especially liked and which Mrs. W. shared with her and sometimes with Mother. I could not visit every day, but I did manage three or four days a week to be there at noon, and the four of us had a kind of picnic. On days when I could not be there, Mrs. W. would encourage Mother to eat. At times Mother could not handle a fork very well, or even a spoon, but she could hold a banana in her hand and she would eat bananas when she would eat nothing else. So I kept the room well-stocked with bananas for all three of them: Mother, her roommate, and Mrs. W.

Across the hall from Mother was a man with Parkinson's disease, whose wife came twice a day, bringing her own meal, to eat with him. She, too, kept an eye on Mother. In return, when she was a few minutes late, I would assure him that she would be there; or if I knew that for some reason she could not come at that time, I would tell him why. In spite of his debilitating disease, he remained a charming gentleman until he died, and I enjoyed knowing him.

A perfect stranger to me, a young woman whose father-in-law was an intermittent patient, always stopped to see my mother when she came to see him. My friends who came to visit other patients also stopped to see Mother; they told me when they had done this, knowing that Mother would not remember their visit, much less tell me, and that it pleased me to know that she was getting attention whether she remembered it or not.

On the whole, the staff at the Extended Care Unit were helpful, though there were some who refused to do anything for a patient who was not assigned to them. Relatives of the patients soon learned who the helpful and cooperative ones were and no doubt we imposed on them, but we tried to express our appreciation to them in whatever small ways we could.

When Mother entered the Extended Care Unit it contained a Skilled Nursing Facility at one end of the corridor and an Intermediate Care Facility at the other end. Mother was in the ICF. Eventually, the hospital decided to convert the entire wing to a Skilled Nursing Facility. Though Mother would have been allowed to remain there, we would have had to pay twice as much as when she was receiving intermediate care. The hospital was considerate enough to raise the rates gradually, but even so the cost was rapidly becoming much more than we could afford. It was time to look for another place for her.

I found a good nursing home about a half-hour's drive from my house, and I was able to visit her at least twice a week. In the summer or during other vacations when I was not teaching, I managed to see her more often. It was in many ways more suitable than the Extended Care Unit had been, and I therefore did not mind the extra time spent in driving.

It is housed in a converted motel and has a homelike quality seldom found in such places. Located in a tiny village of about three hundred people, it attracts both patients and staff members from the surrounding area. The nurses, the administrators, the nurses' aides, the cooks, and the social workers are thus caring for friends and former neighbors, not strangers.

I discovered this little jewel of a nursing home one Sunday afternoon when there was an open house in progress. Friends had told me of the home, but I could not believe that a little hamlet of three hundred people could contain an institution suitable for anyone in my family. It is hard to shake off the snobbishness that results from always living in cities!

As I entered the building, I saw a well-dressed young woman sweeping one of the lounges. I asked her a few questions and learned that she was a social worker. When I expressed surprise at the fact that she was sweeping the floor, she replied, "Out here each of us does whatever needs doing."

It was true. In the Extended Care Facility the emphasis had been on efficiency. One worker brought the dinner trays to the patients' rooms; someone else was responsible for seeing that each tray was placed conveniently for the patient. Sometimes, unfortunately, the second helper did not appear; the result of this "efficiency" then was that though the workers did their jobs quickly, the patients were sometimes neglected. In a less rigidly controlled situation, where each one does "whatever needs doing," the patients are better cared for.

The quality of food is important, as well as the way it is served and the help patients are given in eating it. In each of the institutions where Mother stayed, the food was good, as institutional food goes. Mother never complained about it, and when she did not eat it, it was either because she had no appetite or because she was so unaware of what was going on that she did not notice food placed in front of her.

Before putting anyone into a home it is wise to eat a meal or two there and to observe, as often as possible, the kind of food that the patients are given. Some homes, according to newspaper records, have been found to keep patients on starvation diets. It should be easy to detect such situations by dropping in occasionally at meal time, before placing a patient in the home. If visits are permitted only at specified hours, for example between two and four in the afternoon, and it is not possible to see what kind of food the patients are given or how they are cared for in the mornings and evenings, there is probably more wrong with the place than the food.

It is important, also, to find out what doctors will be taking care of the patient. It may be possible to keep the doctor who has been treating her, but not all doctors will go to a nursing home, and a change may be necessary. In most homes, several doctors are available, so one still has a choice, though limited.

In addition to the three institutions where Mother stayed, I visited several others. I have already described one of these, which over a period of five years changed from a small, pleasant nursing home into an enormous complex, housing a large population of apparently heavily-sedated patients. But nursing homes can change for the better, as well as for the worse.

Not far from my house is a nursing home which has changed management several times. When I first saw the place, shortly before bringing Mother to live with me, I was shocked. It was stark, undecorated, more like a prison than a home for the infirm elderly. All the patients were wearing hospital gowns. Some of them were barefoot, sitting on the cement floor. Others were in wheelchairs, in a room where the sole attendant sat in a corner and seemed to be only slightly more alert than the patients.

Now, however, this same place is pleasant and attractive, with beautiful plants hanging where the patients can see them. The owners, a young couple with children of elementary school age, live on the premises, are genuinely interested in the patients, and do everything possible to make their lives pleasant. Church groups and other organizations are encouraged to visit and hold services or provide entertainment. An activities director does what she can to provide the patients with work in handicrafts. Such activities are typical of good nursing homes. What is not typical, however, is the constant presence of the owners' dog, a collie trained to wander from bed to bed, wheelchair to wheelchair, to be petted by the patients. Many patients who would respond to nothing else have responded to this unusual animal. Unfortunately, when I needed a place for my mother to stay the young couple now managing the home had not yet bought it.

One home which I considered was said to be the best in the state. I was impressed by its cleanliness and its attractiveness. It did not look like a nursing home so much as a hotel or resort. The rooms were spacious and pleasant. The patients, many of them ambulatory, were all dressed in their own clothing. There was a piano, and one of the patients was playing it while I was there. There were magazines on the coffee tables in the lounges. The draperies were elegant, and the potted palms added to the tone of the place. I was impressed, and put Mother's name on the waiting list.

Fortunately, she was accepted in the smaller home—the converted motel—before there was a vacancy in the more elegant one. I was relieved, actually, for three reasons. First, the large home was forty miles from me, the smaller one less than twenty. Second, although Mother loved beautiful surroundings, I had some misgivings about placing her in such a spacious environment, fearing that she would become more disoriented than ever. I envisioned her sitting in one of the lounges, purse in hand, thinking she was waiting for someone to take her home from a hotel. Third, I was not sure that she could meet the standards. When I mentioned to the manager, who was showing me the place, that sometimes Mother ate with her fingers, she replied, "We try to discourage that." I was always delighted when Mother was aware of food set in front of her, and I saw no reason to complain about how she ate it, as long as she ate it. Except for the time she was living with me, getting her to eat was a major problem, and the way she did it seemed trivial.

In a recent television movie, "A Piano for Mrs. Cirino," starring Bette Davis, an ideal nursing home is depicted—better than any one I have seen, and perhaps better than any which actually exist. The patients were treated with kindness and given the attention they needed; there was even an attempt to stimulate their minds with games involving memory. The home was proud of its "graduates"—people who had stayed there and been rehabilitated so that they could return to a more normal lifestyle. Mrs. Cirino, who suffered from depression, not from a true dementia, was one of those graduates, so the film had a happy ending. The fate of the home was less happy, but more believable. It changed management and became just another "warehouse" for putting away the old people, keeping them sedated and hopelessly lost to the real world. In such institutions, which are far too common in our country, the only way to graduate is to die. Conditions in substandard nursing homes have fortunately been publicized in recent years, however, and many have been forced to raise their standards or to go out of business.

Predictions for the future, based on the obvious increase in the older population and the assumption that there is no alternative to placing a large percentage of the elderly in institutions, are generally pessimistic. I believe that there is some evidence, however, that fewer rather than more nursing homes may be needed as research continues in diseases of the middle and older years and as alternatives to insitutional care are increased.

In the first place, the diseases of the elderly, including mental disorders, are receiving more attention by researchers than ever before. Dr. Lewis Thomas, Chancellor of Memorial Sloan-Kettering Cancer Center in New York, maintains in an

article in the January 1984 issue of *Vanity Fair* (pp. 40-41) that
although there is a great deal to be learned about the diseases
of old age, including dementia, much work is being done in
that area. He predicts that in time those of us who live in an
industrial society (he excludes the populations of the developing
countries) can be free of disease for our entire life. In the second
place, it is possible that other social arrangements will be made
which will delay for several years the necessity for placing an
elderly patient in a nursing home.

We have become aware of some of the needs of the elderly,
and some excellent services have become fairly common. Meals
on Wheels is one example; however, it would have helped my
mother only if the person delivering the meal had stayed to see
that she ate it—certainly not possible when there are meals to
be delivered to others. A daily telephone call, while helpful to
many, would probably have confused her. Home health services
might have been somewhat beneficial, if they had been available. But what is most urgently needed, for families who care
for a patient with dementia, is an Adult Day Care Center.

Such Centers have existed in Scandinavian countries and
in the British Commonwealth for years, and are at long last
getting a start in our country. They are still relatively rare,
however, and are not highly publicized. For those of us who
have needed them they have been "America's best kept secret,"
as one clergyman said to me. He was unaware of them, and I
have talked to other clergymen who were surprised to learn of
them. One nurse that I know has visited a Center in Norway,
but has never been in one in the United States. They are hard
to find here.

Adult Day Care Centers are sometimes connected with a
nursing home, where the day patients may mingle with the
fulltime patients, or a hospital; sometimes they are in free-
standing buildings, perhaps near a Senior Citizens Center.
They serve people who are recovering from an illness and need
daily attention after having been dismissed from a hospital;
people from families where everyone works, and where a disabled or elderly person cannot be left alone all day; and people
like my mother, who are too confused to be left alone, but are
still able to walk around and to relate somewhat to other

people.

Physical therapy is usually provided, and the day may start with exercises. A variety of activities is programmed. Often there is music. Transportation to and from the Center is usually provided. The Center is typically open five days a week, from 7:30 to 5. The evidence of the success of the Centers is anecdotal, but convincing. In Melbourne, Australia, one of the patients liked the Center so well that he arrived at five a.m. one Sunday, with his suitcase, and demanded the right to live there. In the United States, a patient who had sat in the corner and cried when he first arrived at the Center eventually "graduated" and returned as a volunteer, leading an exercise group every morning.

We desperately need more Adult Day Care Centers, and the few that we already have need to be highly publicized. Social workers, clergymen, doctors, nurses, and nursing home administrators should know about them, and pressure should be brought on government agencies to see that funding is available.

Meanwhile, as private citizens, we can try to make life as pleasant as possible for friends and relatives who must be kept in nursing homes.

CHAPTER VI

Nursing Homes: How The Patients Can Be Helped

One day after two of my grandchildren and I had visited my mother at the Extended Care Unit, we stopped for a few minutes at the reception desk so that I could ask the head nurse a few questions. When the conversation, which lasted less than ten minutes, was over the children and I walked down the hall to the elevator, where we met a friend who had been visiting several patients. "I just said hello to your mother," she said, "and asked her about you and her great-grandchildren. She told me that she hadn't seen you for ages."

That kind of thing happened often, not only to me but to other visitors. One day I went in Mother's room and said to her roommate, "How is your sister?" "I don't know," she replied, "She never comes to see me." She was speaking of Mrs. W., who came to see her, I knew, every day. When I saw Mrs. W. in the hall a few minutes later I reported the conversation with some amusement. "Well," said Mrs. W. philosophically, "She's entitled to her opinion."

I was sometimes asked by well-meaning friends why I bothered to visit my mother, since she did not even remember that I had been there. The hospital staff assured me, however, that the patients whose families were frequent visitors adjusted much better than those who were left alone. Furthermore, it always seemed to me that a few minutes of personal contact is helpful, even if forgotten immediately.

Some doctors and nursing home staff advise staying away from the patient for a few days at first to give her a chance to adjust. I asked Mother's doctor about the advisability of this and was told to use my own judgement, but that a day or so for adjustment might be beneficial for some patients. Much depends on the individual patient, on the institution, and on the other responsibilities of the visitor.

When I first began visiting Mother in the Extended Care Unit I found it helpful to take someone along with me, as making conversation with her was increasingly difficult. I was fortunate in having several grandchildren, and whenever possible I took two or more of them with me. To keep them amused, I kept coloring books, crayons, puzzles, and other toys in one of Mother's drawers. I would set Mother's adjustable table at the right height so that the children could stand up beside it and color, and Mother, in her wheelchair, enjoyed watching them. The four of us kept up some kind of running conversation; children always have something to talk about. The two little boys especially enjoyed these visits, but Michael and Sarah, as they grew older, seemed bored. I would usually cut their visits a little short, but I did not want to discontinue them entirely. Mother's face always lit up when she saw them, and it doesn't hurt children to be bored occasionally, especially if they are giving pleasure to someone else.

All four children could play the piano a little, and we sometimes rolled Mother in her chair to the lounge, where they would perform briefly. It was not much of a concert from a musical point of view, but the other patients, as well as Mother, seemed to enjoy having children to look at. Occasionally they even applauded. There was a cabinet of toys in the lounge, and with the attendant's permission I sometimes got some of them out for the children to play with. We always put them back carefully before we left.

In a few nursing homes it is permissible to take pets. This could not have been allowed in the hospital-like atmosphere of the Extended Care Unit, but I know of less formal institutions where well-behaved dogs on a leash are welcome, though taking one at meal-time cannot be permitted.

When I did not have the children with me I frequently rolled Mother's chair into other rooms to visit with patients I knew. One was the woman who had taken care of Mother on Essie's day off. She was in the Skilled Nursing Facility down the hall from Mother. Although in extremely poor health, she enjoyed company and seeing my mother as well as me. Another patient was the mother of one of the doctors. A former teacher of German, she was fond of poetry, both German and English. So occasionally I would take a book of poems with me—English, of course—and read to her. I do not know how much she comprehended, as her mind was not always clear, but she liked having someone come into the room and read to her. Mother, on the other hand, enjoyed this activity much less than watching the children with their color crayons, so I limited the poetry-reading sessions to ten minutes or so.

There was one patient in her nineties, less disoriented than most, who liked to play checkers. At times I would take Mother into this patient's room and play a game with her, and Mother did not seem to mind watching us. The game never lasted long, perhaps because my opponent cheated a lot. I ignored the cheating politely, but once she scolded me for not catching her. For her, cheating was part of the challenge; it wasn't fun if no one tried to catch her at it. When I learned this, I began accusing her when she cheated, and she found the game more interesting.

Mother became progressively less aware of her surroundings. Her sister flew up to visit once or twice a year, for a few days, and I took her to see Mother every day. One day when I had some errands to do I left her with Mother. She had brought some sewing with her, and sat in Mother's room with her handiwork. When I returned an hour or so later, she was in the room by herself.

"Where is Mother?" I asked in surprise.

"She said she had to go see about something," my aunt replied. I went to the lounge to look for her, and found her sitting idly at a table. Obviously she had forgotten about her visitor, if indeed she had even realized when she left her room that she had one. My aunt, understanding Mother's condition, was not offended. We were both amused.

Many people dread visiting nursing homes and hospitals, but such visits need not be depressing, especially if one feels that they are helpful to others. The staff at the Extended Care Unit were efficient, but often short-handed, and we visitors did what we could to help patients, especially at mealtime. Down the hall from Mother was a woman who could feed herself most of what was on her plate but could not manage the slippery jello she was sometimes given for dessert. As one of us passed by her door, she would call out, and we would go in and feed her. It was not a time-consuming chore as she ate fast. Helping my mother with a meal, on the other hand, could take over an hour.

For a while Mother shared her room with Miss T., an elderly lady who was the sister of the president of my bank. Her brother and his wife came fairly often to see her and to keep her clothes in order. Both she and my mother were still ambulatory at the time, and both dressed themselves every day, with some help from the staff. Once in a while Mother would put on something that belonged to Miss T., who was a large woman, and Mother then looked rather pathetic in a dress several sizes too big for her. But Miss T. never objected.

When Mother became weaker and unable to walk, as she did after about three years in an institution, I noticed that sometimes she was wearing a dress turned backward. All her dresses buttoned down the front, and I finally realized that the helpers who dressed her found it easier to slip them on and off her, when she was in a wheelchair, if they put them on her backwards. It was a practical solution to a problem but the result looked rather strange.

When my aunt saw Mother dressed in that fashion she volunteered to take her dresses and cut them open down the back, putting ties at the neck, so that they could be slipped onto mother when she was sitting down. After this was done Mother certainly looked more comfortable.

While she could walk I took Mother to the beauty parlor once a week, as I had taken her when she was living with me. When she became weaker and spent more time in a wheelchair and the trips seemed to cause more disorientation, her beauty operator went to the Extended Care Unit from time to time to wash and set her hair. I would have been glad to pay someone to manicure her fingernails, and her toenails too, if possible, but I could find no one in our community with both the skill and the time to supply that service. Some nursing homes have beauty parlors, usually with a beautician who comes once a week; Fran, who did Mother's hair, was not employed by the Extended Care Facility, but she did use the beauty parlor there when she went to shampoo and set Mother's hair. At the last nursing home where Mother lived there was a similar arrangement, with a beautician who lived nearby, but there was some problem about state licensing. Much to the distress of the management, their beauty parlor could not be used very often.

Every institution for people in Mother's condition should have a beauty parlor available for the patients at least once a week. The more services offered the better: shampoos and sets, manicures, pedicures, even facials. I have noticed that well-groomed patients are more outgoing than patients who are simply showered (sometimes quite hastily) and dried off, as if they were non-people.

By the time Mother was moved to her last nursing home she was unable to walk at all. She had had pneumonia several times, and she was weaker after each recovery. But almost until the end she was able to sit up in a wheelchair, and keeping her attractively dressed and well-groomed made a difference.

Just as I had enjoyed getting to know members of the staff, some of the other patients, and the people who came to visit them at the Extended Care Unit, I soon became acquainted with the staff and other patients at Mother's new residence. Since this place was not in the town where I lived I knew fewer of the visitors. Some of the patients, however, were mentally alert, especially those who suffered from physical problems rather than chronic brain disorders, and I became friends with them.

Mother's roommate was just about as confused as Mother was, but she liked to talk. Mrs. S. had a large Bible which she held constantly on her lap, reading over and over the inscription on the fly-leaf: "To Mom, with love, Easter 1978." This gift seemed to give her unending pleasure, and every time I went to see Mother, Mrs. S. told me that she had just found it. She also told me many times about where she had lived as a child, between a church and a school house. We sometimes talked about gardens, and I told her what I had planted or harvested. I never tired of her response to my "How are you today, Mrs. S.?"

"I'm here but bein' keerful," she invariably replied.

I enjoyed getting to know the patients and talking with them, trying to bring Mother into the conversation as much as possible, with little success. It was almost as if she had said everything that she needed to say and was no longer interested in talking. But she liked the buzz of conversation around her, I believe.

The patient I most enjoyed talking with at this home was Doris C., who was completely lucid but quite handicapped physically. She was confined to a wheelchair, as she had been all her life; her arms and legs were twisted in such a way that she had little use of them, though she could feed herself. I tried to do little things for Doris; for example, when she expressed a wish to listen to the Bible on tapes (it was hard for her to turn the pages of a book), I borrowed the complete set of the Old Testament and took it to her, one or two tapes at a time, until she had listened to them all.

Doris took an interest in my mother and always told me when she had appeared to be relaxed and contented. It was a comfort to me to know that Doris was nearby to speak to Mother and to smile at her occasionally. We became good friends.

When I felt compelled to visit my mother several times a week, it often seemed a chore, and it never occurred to me that after her death I would go back to such institutions voluntarily. But I do. After several years, I am no longer unduly upset by the condition of the patients, and I actually enjoy talking with some of them.

I have found that friends are sometimes willing to go with me. Once, when Mother was still alive, a young nursing student, who had emigrated from Thailand and was attending our college, asked to go along. The patients adored her. She would kneel down beside their wheelchairs so that her face was level with theirs, and their response to her was beautiful. One patient, who had had several strokes and was unable to speak, kept making strange noises which I could not understand. When I got a nurse to come and see what she wanted, I learned that she wanted the Thai student to come over and talk to her. Of course the young woman went promptly to her, and the patient's face lit up with joy.

I know a young housewife who sets aside each Thursday for a "visiting day," when she goes to see patients in hospitals and nursing homes. She used to drop in to see Mother's roommate, whom she knew, and she always had a few cheerful words for Mother as well. The world needs more people like her.

Many organizations make it a practice to do things for people in institutions. Churches arrange for Sunday afternoon services. Schoolchildren sometimes go to sing songs or present other entertainment. At Christmas, especially, groups of children and adults visit the patients and sing carols, with the patients sometimes joining in. All this is helpful.

But most helpful of all, I believe, are visits from people who go often enough and stay long enough to get to know the patients. The visitors benefit perhaps as much as the patients. For probably there is nowhere else that one can find so many examples of courage, forbearance, and heroic acceptance of one's fate.

CHAPTER VII

If Only . . .

When a ninety-seven-year-old woman fell and broke her arm, the daughter with whom she was living was guilt-ridden. "If we had put her in a nursing home," she said ruefully, "this wouldn't have happened."

Maybe not, but something else might have. She might, for example, have become extremely depressed. Possibly she would have become bedridden. Which is better, to be bedridden and depressed or ambulatory with a broken arm? The trouble is that the elderly person, especially if she has any form of dementia, cannot make her own decisions. Those of us who are or have been responsible for such a person can never say, "It's her own fault." We feel that whatever happens is *our* fault.

If we put an elderly relative in a nursing home, we often feel guilty, even though we visit her often and do everything possible to provide for her comfort. If we keep her at home, however, and she is unhappy or disturbs the household, we may feel equally guilty.

At times we may also feel—in addition to guilt—anger, helplessness, embarrassment, fear, and grief. We will probably feel some of these emotions when caring for anyone who is incapacitated, even temporarily. When the problem is dementia such feelings are more intense, for the patient cannot make any decisions for herself. It is fruitless to discuss living and care-taking arrangements with a person who cannot remember or understand what is being discussed.

I realize now that I could have had such a discussion when Mother's early symptoms of dementia began, especially when she complained to me of her loss of memory and I dismissed her complaints as trivial. Most of us have experienced walking into a room and not being able to remember why we went there or what we wanted to get. This was the kind of memory lapse I thought my mother was talking about—this, and other such common phenomena as temporarily forgetting someone's name, or being unable to think of a certain word. We all have had such words "on the tip of the tongue." I thought nothing of Mother's apprehensions, and usually dismissed them with a reference to a woman we knew who was then living in a retirement center and who was truly confused and forgetful. "You're fine," I would say to my mother. "Now if you were as forgetful as Margaret, we would really have something to worry about."

In less than a year Mother was in a condition worse than Margaret's. She had had cause to worry, and I had been wrong to dismiss her worries. I had assumed that she had another fifteen or twenty years to live, which she did have, and that they would be enjoyable years, which they were not. I still have to keep reminding myself that even if I had known the seriousness of the situation, probably nothing could have been done about it, except that Mother and I could have talked about her future. Maybe. I do not know exactly how we would have approached such a discussion, or whether or not it would have been fruitful. But I have felt guilty because I was not astute enough to recognize her condition.

I have also felt guilty about going over three thousand miles away from her, to a new job. I live only a ten-hour drive from the city where many of our relatives live, and I was disappointed when she refused to move there and be near them. Even though I still thought that she was in good mental and physical health, I realized that she should not stay so far from all her family when she was approaching old age, even a normal and healthy old age. Her sisters were eager for her to return to their home city. She had innumerable friends and other relatives there, and although she had not spent a winter there in over forty years, she had gone "home," as we still called it, just about every other summer, and friends and relatives from there had frequently visited her.

Less than a year after I left, she was too confused and disoriented to travel alone. When her sister and brother-in-law went for her, they had to take complete charge of her and her affairs.

So I have felt more guilt because I did not go and get her myself. It would have been extremely difficult, leaving a new teaching position for a couple of weeks the very first year, but I could have managed it. The truth is, however, that I was not at all sure that my going would do any good; I was afraid that if I went, I would have to stay there and take care of her.

As an only child, I always expected to take care of my mother in her old age, but I did not expect her to become old so suddenly. Within less than a year she seemed to become an old woman, and *I had to decide what to do about her.* Our extended family has always been very close, so when the crisis occurred and I was taken unawares, I looked to my aunts—her sisters— for a solution. They made suggestions and were helpful in many ways, but I realized with a shock that I had to make the final decision. The responsibility was mine and I was not prepared for it.

I accepted the responsibility, but not with as much inward grace as I might have. I knew that my own life would be disrupted even more than it had been when I had small children to care for. I never resented the time I spent taking care of the children, as I looked forward to a future when they would be able to take care of themselves, and I felt that preparing them for that future was a constructive activity.

But what is constructive about taking care of an old person who needs attention as much as or even more than a small child? The only future for such a person is death. I began to feel resentment—not against my mother, who certainly had not been responsible for our situation—but against the turn my life had taken. I resented having to spend time at home when I wanted to be somewhere else—in my office, at the library, at a friend's house, or at a meeting. When I had to be away from home, aside from the regular routine of classes and office hours, I felt as if I were being pulled in two directions, or sometimes four—like a prisoner who is being executed by having each limb tied to a horse, and the four horses driven in different directions. The image is a grim one, but to my shame, that is the way I often felt: grim, bitter, and resentful. And I felt guilty because of my resentment and bitterness.

Mother had been with me only a month when a colleague

at the university where I had formerly taught called me long distance, asking me to join her at the National Council of Teachers of English meeting in Atlanta at Thanksgiving. How could I? I told her, with despair and resignation in my voice, that I would never be able to attend a professional meeting again. My reaction was no doubt extreme. Although Essie was then staying with us, she did not drive a car and she was unfamiliar with the town, having lived in it only a little over a month. I did not see how I could leave Mother and Essie alone, in a strange place, with no transportation.

But my friend was persistent, and urged me to try to work something out. I found that Essie's Thursday replacement, who lived only a few blocks away, was willing to stay with Mother for several days. So I not only went to the meeting; I also took Essie along so that she could visit cousins in Atlanta for a couple of days.

After that, I believe that I no longer felt resentful. How could I, when relatives were willing to have Mother visit them, when they often came to our home to see us and help me with her, and when friends later offered to stay with her while I went to meetings and sometimes even while I was away on a trip?

When I convinced myself that I was doing everything possible for Mother, I felt guilty about my work. At a small college one is expected to spend a great deal of time with individual students, to get to know them and to give them as much help as possible. The first year that I taught at the college, before Mother came to live with me, I had been able to do that. After she arrived, however, I was no longer free to stay late in my office to talk to students. I met all my classes, had as many individual conferences as I could manage, and made preparations and graded papers conscientiously. I often brought work home with me, which is certainly not unusual for a teacher. What was unusual was that I graded papers or made preparations after I had gone to bed at night, so that Mother would assume that I was asleep and would not interrupt me. I learned to keep books and papers under the covers, so that if she did wander into my room she would think I was just about to turn off the light.

Even so, I never felt that I had enough time to spend working in the library or talking with students in my office. When Essie was with us, I often stayed until five; but there were times when I needed to go back in the evening, and I hated to leave Mother. Essie was not enough; Mother wanted me. When we had less efficient help, the situation was even harder.

After five years of having my mother at home, trying to make her comfortable and contented, even planting flowers where she could see them through the glass doors leading to the patio, I felt that I had tried everything, and I arranged for her to be admitted to the Extended Care Unit. Then I really felt guilty.

Some people can, apparently, put an elderly relative away in a home and never go back to see her. Such people seem to have solved the problem, and their consciences seem to be clear. For most of us, however, the matter is less simple. At first, just walking through a nursing home, even a well-run one, is depressing. Even if we do not know the people in wheelchairs or walkers, who sometimes reach out and say to strangers, "Please take me home" or "Get me out of here," we feel guilt. After all, we have been taught that we are our brothers' (and our parents') keepers. Our consciences remind us that their last years should be spent with dignity, surrounded by a loving family.

When we can't make this happen we blame ourselves. Even if we keep the person at home we feel guilty: about the patient, who is not happy, and about the rest of the family, who may be neglected, inconvenienced, and sometimes embarrassed.

Women are especially vulnerable. Dr. Matti Gershenfeld, director of the Couples Learning Center in Jenkintown, Pennsylvania, has noted the remarks heard frequently from her women clients: "I feel so guilty all the time—about my kids, my job, my husband, and my mother."[1] According to Carol Gilligan, Associate Professor of Education at Harvard, women are more susceptible to guilt feelings than are men.[2]

Men are not free of such feelings, however. A young college professor has told me that he cannot even think of his parents, who are still comparatively young and in good physical and mental health, without feeling guilty. His reason? He has managed to procure for himself a better education than they had.

It helps, I believe, to remember that others also feel guilty. Lynne Steinman, a therapist at Ingleside Mental Center in Rosemead, California, says:

> The adult children I talk to most often are the ones whose parents are in transition from an acute hospital to a convalescent hospital. Their parent has had a stroke, and their major problem is guilt. They say things like, 'If only I had gotten her to a hospital earlier,' 'If only I had kept her house cleaner so she wouldn't have tripped over that light cord,' 'If only I had watched her diet more carefully and not let her eat so much salt.'
>
> They so often feel that they haven't done enough and they have usually done too much. They want to win approval of their parents and in many cases they never had it and are never going to get it. Many of them historically had a tenuous relationship all along with the parent.[3]

Article after article, by specialists and laymen, attest to the prevalence of guilt feelings among people who care for the ill and aged. Patricia Archbold, who has made a careful study of middle-aged people caring for their parents, is quoted as saying, "Despite the obvious sacrifices children make to nurse such parents, the single most common feeling is guilt."[4] Knowing their parents have had a hard life, she says, "They feel there's nothing they could do that would be enough to make up for that." If they pay others to care for their parent, they feel guilty about their "lack of time and lack of energy to meet the competing demands of their parent, children, husband and work."[5]

The problem with most of us may be that we are "moral climbers"; the term, analogous to *social climbers*, is used by Theodor Reik in his book *Myth and Guilt: the Crime and Punishment of Mankind*. A moral climber, Reik says, is a person who tries to live beyond a normal moral standard, and who makes "energetic, sometimes even desperate efforts to mount to a moral position that is too high, compared to his means and abilities."[6]

Ann Landers, in an article written for *Family Circle* (Sept. 1978), while noting the heroic qualities of people who care for ill or elderly parents at home, adds "This can be the most physically exhausting and emotionally draining job in the world. I implore children not to feel guilty if they are unable to do it."

I never found time to write to Ann Landers or to Dear Abby, but I have been comforted by their answers to other people in circumstances similar to mine. I realize now that my guilt feelings were (and still are) triggered by everything I did, and—paradoxically—by everything I failed to do. No doubt they were caused to a great extent by my trying to be a "moral climber." In retrospect, here is the list of actions for which I felt (and sometimes still feel) guilty.

I should have paid more attention to my mother and shown more concern for her in the early stages of her illness, when her deviance from normal behavior was minimal. I should have been more alert.

I should not have tried to pass the buck, to arrange for her to live in a nursing home near her sisters instead of with me. I did not, as I could have, consent to her living *with* them, as I felt that that would be too hard on them. But was I right? My mother was happier with them than she was with me.

I should not have moved away from her when she was seventy-six years old.

When the people I employed to stay with her and care for her did not please her, I should have quit my job and stayed with her myself. She would have liked that.

I should have tried harder to keep her busy and entertained.

When I put her in an institution, her needs and comfort were sometimes neglected. I should have kept her at home.

I should have visited her every day when she was in the Extended Care Unit or in a nursing home.

I should have spent less time with her than I did and more time having individual conferences with my students.

It is obvious from this account that most of my guilt feelings were caused by confusion, by not knowing the "best" thing to do. The most helpful advice that I have read for handling such guilt feelings is given by Dr. Gershenfeld, who recommends substituting other terms for the word *guilt*. We should avoid the word *guilty,* she says, for it is judgmental and has a permanence to it, and substitute terms such as *confused, unsure about priorities, sad, worried, concerned.*[7] Each of these terms is applicable, at times, to those of us caring for a person with dementia. I have taken these terms and applied them to our situation.

We are confused, because the patient is confused. We can seldom communicate coherently with her. We do not know what is best for her and for the other family members.

We are unsure about priorities. Is it better to keep the patient at home, sometimes at the expense of disrupting the household, or to put her in a nursing home, which is seldom best for her but often permits a more wholesome atmosphere for others concerned?

We are sad. No matter what we do, we can seldom, if ever, bring happiness to a person whose mind is diseased. She is sad, and we share her sadness. In a few cases she may be contented, perhaps even happy, with her daydreams, as was the woman described in this letter:[8]

> I pity those who are ill and suffer with pain, but a lot of those old folks are like my Mom. They don't suffer—they are senile. Very little of their minds are left.
>
> These are the people who reach out to you as you walk down the hall. Don't pity them because they look bored and appear to have no interest in life. They live in a world that is very interesting to them.
>
> My mom sits in a chair doing nothing, but she isn't in that chair at all. She is years away, visiting with her mother, or perhaps she's out to a dance. One day she may be playing with her sister or brother. The next day she may be raising her family. Then again, she may be doing her homework, even cutting up Fels Naptha soap.
>
> Far-fetched? The last time I left her room she said happily, "I'm going to visit Mama's today. We're going to have cookies and milk."
>
> I replied, "Enjoy yourself—and say hello to Grandma."
>   —An Only Daughter

Ann Landers adds that "the authorities on senility say the world these folks live in is the only world they know." I do not know what "authorities" she has read; I have read others with a different opinion, who stress the importance of "reality orientation." Furthermore, I have seen and heard patients, my mother included, who shifted rapidly from illusion to reality. The widow who said, "My husband is coming to get me, and we are going to move to a new apartment," when she was in a nursing home, unable to do anything for herself, said at another time to one of the nurse's aides, "All you people think that because we are old we don't know what is going on around here. We know a lot more than you give us credit for."

I believe her!

So we are sad, and we should be. Dementia is nothing to be joyful about.

We are also worried. Will the patient hurt herself? How much longer will she live? Will her (or our) money last?

We are also concerned: about her comfort, her living arrangements, her emotions, her safety, her (or our) finances.

If we think in terms of our confusion, our sadness, our worry, and our concern, perhaps we will blame ourselves less. Few people can eradicate guilt feelings entirely, as irrational as they sometimes are; they are part of our humanity. But if we become obsessed with guilt we will be in need of as much help as our patient is.

Nor can we expect the feeling of guilt to go away completely after the patient dies. Probably there will always be a trace of it left to haunt us. It is the price we pay for caring.

Notes to Chapter VII

1. Wendy Davis, (pseudonym for Sally Wendkos Olds) "Guilt: Modern Woman's Old-Fashioned Burden," *Ladies Home Journal,* July 1981, p. 26

2. *Ibid.,* p. 28

3. Jane Estes, "Caring for Elderly Parents Can Be Trying Experience for Grown Kids," Knight-Ridder News Service, Pasadena, California. In *Lexington Herald,* Lexington, Kentucky, Sept. 8, 1981, p. C 3

4. Susan Ager, Sunday *Herald-Leader,* Lexington, Kentucky, Nov. 1, 1981, p. E 7

5. *Ibid.*

6. Theodor Reik, *Myth and Guilt: the Crime and Punishment*

of Mankind. New York: George Braziller, Inc., 1957

7. Wendy Davis, p. 28

8. Ann Landers, published in the Open Forum of the La Salle, Illinois News-Tribune and reprinted in Ann Landers' column.

CHAPTER VIII

Financial and Legal Matters

Several years before I realized that my mother was the victim of a serious mental condition, I noticed a change in the way she handled her checking account. She postponed writing checks until after she had received her monthly statement. Apparently she relied on the statement for her balance, rather than on her checkbook.

In some people this would make sense. I have friends who do not even try to balance their accounts, and if I could keep a large reserve in mine, I would be tempted to use this system myself. It has taken me about forty years to become reasonably efficient at handling finances. Obviously I am not qualified to write with authority about financial matters, and I have no serious intentions of doing so. Instead, I am going to make suggestions that may be helpful to others who share my deficiency.

My mother was not one of those people; she had always handled economic affairs with aplomb. When she became aware that she was losing this ability, she refrained from paying her bills until after her bank statement arrived, so that she would have no checks outstanding and could record the statement balance in her checkbook.

By the time we discovered the seriousness of her condition, she had not only stopped writing checks; she had also stopped recording deposits. With the help of the accounting department at her bank, my uncle balanced her checkbook and brought unpaid bills back to me when he and my aunt returned to his home with her. Fortunately, because of provisions which Mother had made almost forty years earlier, I was able to pay the bills myself, writing checks on her account.

Since the time I was in college her bank account had been in my name as well as hers. She considered this arrangement a kind of insurance for me in case of emergency. I used it only when told to do so—for example, when directed to buy myself a present. When she became unable to handle her own affairs, it was no trouble at all for me to take over. This was one advantage of being an only child. With several children she would not have been able to share her account. But even if my name had not already been on her checks, we could have arranged with little or no difficulty to open a joint account.

When several people are responsible for someone in my mother's state of health, it would be wise to select one to take care of finances. I have heard of situations in which the parent, though unable to handle her own affairs, was unwilling to entrust one of her grown children with them. If the parent can be declared incompetent, someone can take over, with or without her consent. It may be advisable to assign the responsibility to someone outside the family—her lawyer, for example. At one time I considered asking our lawyer to take charge of Mother's money, thinking that she might feel more secure about it. There was so little to be done, however, that I decided such a solution would be impractical. I accepted the responsibility myself with misgiving and little confidence, but it was not as formidable as I had expected it to be.

At least there was no family friction which sometimes occurs. Mother's sisters may have disagreed with me and with each other about the best way to take care of her, but no one considered sharing the responsibility for her money with me. When I asked him, my uncle gave me advice on investing the money which she had obtained from the sale of her house, and I followed it.

I invested her money in two Savings and Loan companies, which at the time paid comparatively good interest. Times have changed since 1970, however, and no doubt money could be put to better use in some other way today. Even then, the interest on her savings certificates was less than it would have been had I invested it in something else, but I felt that certificates were safe. More lucrative investments, such as public utilities stocks or money market certificates, would have required me to keep a wary eye on them. I was looking for security, not high profits.

I was careful not to touch her capital, at least at first. Later, I did use some of it for a down payment on a house which my son and his family were living in, but the rent they paid far exceeded the interest Mother was getting on savings certificates.

I have known people to use a parent's capital to pay her expenses, thus making the parent eligible for Medicaid. I have known of other people who transferred all of the parent's assets to their own name, so that she would be eligible for Medicaid.* I am glad that I never felt obliged to do this, though when inflation caused her expenses to double, I thought that I might have to do something of the sort. It was not conscience alone which kept me from using her capital or transferring it to my name. There were several other reasons.

First, if she had been on Medicaid I would have had a limited choice of nursing homes to consider putting her in. Not only would the home have to be approved by a government agency, it would also have to be willing to take Medicaid patients. Many homes prefer "private pay" patients, and some refuse to take those on Medicaid.

Second, I had a vested interest in keeping her capital. As an only child, I would inherit what was left of it when she died; it seemed foolish and unnecessary to use the principal.

Third, it was a considerable comfort to me to have a fairly large sum of money for a possible emergency. When emergencies did arise, however, instead of dipping into the capital I borrowed on the savings certificates, always paying back the loan as quickly as possible.

I have talked with people who used their parent's capital to pay her expenses, expecting her to die within a year or so, and who were in serious financial difficulties when the parent lived for many years. These were not people looking for help from Medicaid; rather, they wanted to give their parent the very best of everything during what they thought would be the last few months of her life.

Once Mother's money was invested, managing her finances was a relatively simple procedure. At first her income was

*Federal legislation passed in 1982 requires a person whose resources are taken over by a relative to wait two years before collecting Supplemental Security Income (SSI) and consequently Medicaid. (People with incomes less than $324.30 a month are eligible for SSI.) This ruling does not affect people who are not eligible for SSI but are still unable to pay their medical expenses.

adequate and her needs were simple. I arranged to have her social security check and her state pension check deposited directly in our joint account, in which I kept her money only. My own income was deposited in another account. Mother received interest every three months on her savings certificates, and I deposited that also in the joint account as it came in. On her occasional visits to see her sisters she took a checkbook with her and, under their supervision, sometimes wrote checks when they took her shopping. She made no attempt to keep a balance, and often did not even write the amount of the check on the stub, but since the checks she wrote were never for a large amount this did not create a great problem. I made necessary adjustments when her bank statement came.

Eventually, because of inflation and the need to put her in a nursing home, her income did not quite cover her expenses. In 1970 the cost of the nursing home where she stayed for a short time had been a little over four hundred dollars a month; in 1980, when she died, the cost of the home where she was staying was about nine hundred. If she had remained in the Extended Care Facility, which was being gradually converted into a Skilled Nursing Facility only, the cost would have exceeded fifteen hundred dollars a month.

My major problem in handling Mother's money was not in making ends meet. It was, especially for the five years she lived with me, calming her fears about what was happening to her money and her concern about its source. Although she had always seemed to have faith in my integrity, she had less confidence in my ability to keep records. She would periodically insist on going over her accounts, making me explain every deposit and every withdrawal again and again. "Where did that money come from?" she would ask repeatedly of every deposit entered. Strangely enough, she seemed less concerned about the withdrawals. I learned to keep her checkbook and bank statements out of sight most of the time, and as the years passed she asked to see them less often. During her last five years when she was in institutions, she showed no interest in finances or, sadly in anything else.

The fact that most of my life I had lived near my mother made it easier for me to take over her affairs than if we had been living a great distance apart. I was familiar with or had

easy access to information about the things that, according to
A. Reading Van Doren, Jr., a New York lawyer, anyone responsible for a senile person needs to know:

the person's source of income, including pensions
her social security number
insurance policies (property, life, health)
safe deposit box—and where the key is kept
whether there is a will, and where it is
names of accountants, brokers, and lawyers if any
rent or mortgage payments
debts owed or money due
papers pertaining to property, such as house or car[1]

Van Doren also mentions getting a power of attorney,
usually a necessary step when taking over someone else's
affairs. This is an uncomplicated procedure, requiring only a
simple form to be signed by the person granting it, and
notarized. The form is available at stationery stores, but it is
also possible to get one in a lawyer's office. Since dementia
progresses rather slowly, and in its early stages the patient
has periods of lucidity (especially in the early morning), taking
care of such business matters is not a serious problem. But it is
extremely important to take care of them as soon as possible,
for eventually the patient may not even be able to sign her
name.

Since legally I was co-owner of my mother's home, and
when it was put up for sale I was not in the city where she was
living, I gave my own power of attorney to her real estate
agent, who happened to be a good friend. This was a restricted
power of attorney, enabling him to sell the house and take care
of all related legal details requiring my signature. When my
mother came back to stay briefly with my aunt and uncle, and
I joined her at their home, I obtained a power of attorney which
enabled me to sign *any* legal document for her. Actually, she
was still able to sign her own name and did sign it to the will
which she made (to replace an older one), but later on it was
necessary for me to take care of all transactions for her.

Even if a person already has made a will, it is wise to have
it reviewed at the onset of dementia—or of what might be
dementia. Making a will is a simple procedure and can be done
without a lawyer, but this can be risky. Bruce Fried, staff

member of the National Senior Citizens' Law Center, says: "It is now so inexpensive to have a will drawn that it doesn't really make sense not to do it. Problems that can be created later for heirs by people trying to save $50 or $100 don't make it worthwhile."[2]

As it turned out, even though Mother's will was only ten years old when she died, a problem occurred. The people who had witnessed the signing of the will were employees of the lawyer who had drawn it up. The lawyer died before my mother did, and the witnesses were no longer employed by his law firm. Eventually I got in touch with the lawyer's widow, who in turn located one of the witnesses. Probably the will would have been considered valid even without locating a witness, but settling Mother's estate would no doubt have taken longer. I should have selected witnesses with more care, from among people I knew.

Where is the best place to keep a will? In a safe deposit box it will be protected from fire or flood or theft or from being misplaced. In most states, however, there are laws pertaining to the opening of a safe deposit box after the death of the renter. Mother's box was in my name as well as hers, but even so, after her death I did not have immediate access to it. Fortunately I had a copy of the will at home.

There are some rights and responsibilities which the next of kin has, regarding the comfort and safety of the patient, which do not require even a power of attorney. For my mother I chose comfort rather than safety, since I felt that the risk to her was minimal.

When I learned that she was being strapped in her bed at night at the Extended Care Unit and that she pleaded every night with the attendant not to strap her in, I went immediately to talk with the head nurse. I understood the reason for the restraints; if Mother had fallen out of bed I could have sued the institution. All I had to do was to sign a paper releasing the hospital from blame should Mother fall and be injured. The head nurse and I agreed that the sides of the bed should be raised, but no restraints were to be used. When Mother moved to the nursing home I made the same arrangements. Although I believe that these arrangements were appropriate for Mother, they might not be wise for all patients.

As a matter of fact, Mother did fall out of bed several times during the last ten years of her life: a couple of times in her own home when her sister was there to help her back into bed; once in the Extended Care Unit; and later in the last nursing home where she stayed, when she hit her head on a bedside table as she fell—the only time that she was injured by falling. It was not a serious injury and required only a bandaid.

When Mother first came to live with me I borrowed a hospital bed with sides that could be raised for her protection. After a few weeks I had to decide whether to return the bed or to buy it, so I consulted her doctor who advised letting her use an ordinary bed.

"Isn't there danger of her falling out and breaking a hip?" I asked, having heard often of elderly people who had fallen and broken a hip.

"Old people's hips break," the doctor explained, "and that is *why* they fall."

I felt that Mother's hip could not possibly break and cause her to fall while she was in bed. Furthermore, if she did fall she was in less danger of injuring herself than a heavy person would probably be. Mother weighed less than a hundred pounds.

In order further to protect her comfort in the Extended Care Unit and, later, in the nursing home, I discussed with her doctors what measures should be taken if she became dangerously ill. My desire, I explained to them, was to have her kept comfortable, not to have her life prolonged by mechanical measures which would perhaps be painful to her. I believe in death with dignity, and I was certain that Mother would have requested such a death had she been able to make a choice. Every doctor who took care of her agreed with me that in her case, heroic measures to prolong her life should not be taken. She was given intravenous feedings on a few occasions when she contracted pneumonia, but that was simply to help her regain her strength more rapidly. It was not what I would consider a heroic measure.

Arranging for a checking account, making deposits or having checks assigned to the bank, paying bills, obtaining power of attorney, having a will drawn up, and taking legal responsibility for the patient's comfort—all these procedures are fairly easy to take care of. One other responsibility, however, requires considerable red tape. For me, requesting reimbursement from Mother's health insurance was a dreaded chore.

She had three policies: Medicare, Medical Indemnity of of America (MIA), and Colonial Penn. She had taken out the Colonial Penn policy several years before she retired, and though it was expensive (over nineteen dollars a month), I was reluctant to drop it, as I felt that she would not want me to do so. The MIA policy was part of her retirement package.

While Mother was living with me and when she was in the Extended Care Unit her medical bills were no problem, as the two doctors who took care of her were connected with the college where I was teaching and were paid a salary by that institution. Since Mother was not financially dependent on me, I was surprised that these doctors were willing to take care of her. When I asked one of them if he would do so, it was because I felt that he and his colleague on the college staff were excellent doctors and because he consented to make house calls if necessary.

"People who take care of elderly parents at home," he said kindly, "deserve all the help they can get."

Because neither of these doctors was permitted to charge for services, I was spared the experience of filling out Medicare forms for physician's bills, covered by Part B of Medicare. On the few occasions when Mother was transferred, because of brief illness, from the Extended Care Unit to the main part of the hospital, requests for reimbursement for Part A of Medicare (hospital insurance) had to be submitted, but the hospital sent in the request and also submitted the forms for her Colonial Penn insurance. The MIA forms had to be submitted by the patient, so I had to take care of those for her.

After Mother was moved to another nursing home, too far away for the college doctors to visit her, I had to assume more responsibility for collecting from Medicare and her other policies. The year before Mother died, I became eligible for Medicare myself. Keeping track of expenses and filling out forms for both of us was a task I did not enjoy.

Now that I no longer have to take care of Mother's health claims, just my own, I feel that I am beginning to understand how to do it. A useful guide, published by Collier-Macmillan in 1981, is *How to Recover Your Medical Expenses: A Compre-*

hensive Guide to Understanding and Unscrambling Medicare.
Written by Ken Waller, this inexpensive book covers not only
Medicare claims, but supplemental insurance and medical tax
deductions.

Although Medicare benefits are subject to change, some
basic facts seem likely to remain constant:

1. Medicare Part A is hospital insurance. It pays part of
hospital expenses, including part of the costs of after-hospital
care in a skilled nursing facility or at home.

2. Medicare Part B is medical insurance. It helps pay doctor
bills, bills for medical services, and the cost of some medical
supplies, such as wheelchairs and crutches.

Almost everyone over sixty-five is covered by Medicare.
Some people are covered also by Medicaid, a public assistance
program for qualified people regardless of age. The following
people qualify for this public assistance program:

1. Recipients of Supplemental Security Income (SSI)

2. Recipients of Aid to Families with Dependent Children
(AFDC)

3. Recipients of aid to low-income aged, blind, and disabled
people.

More specific, current, and complete information on Medicare can be obtained at any Social Security Office. Information
on Medicaid can be obtained at a local social services department, often called the Department of Human Resources.
Addresses for these agencies can be found in telephone direc-
tories. Hospitals and nursing homes usually have a social service worker who will also be helpful if it seems advisable to ask
for Medicaid for a patient. The administrator of a nursing home
is another person to consult.

Although Mother was never on Medicaid, if she had lived
much longer I might have had to request it. When she died, her
monthly income was about two hundred dollars less than her
expenses, and I was paying the difference. I was on the verge
of retirement, however, and not certain that I would be able to
continue that much financial help, especially if her expenses
kept increasing. A social service worker explained to me that
her income from Social Security, her state pension, and interest

on savings certificates would be used to pay as much of her nursing home expenses as possible, and Medicaid would supplement that. This arrangement would result in her paying a daily rate at the nursing home that was slightly less than she was currently paying, as the government paid less than private patients were charged. I talked with the owner and supervisor of the nome, who assured me that Mother would be permitted to stay there at this reduced rate. (When I asked her if I could slip her the difference under the table, she looked at me askance. Probably such a deal would have landed us both in jail!)

Since Mother died the same month that I retired, I nevei had to make the decision to request Medicaid for her.

Often physicians will file the Medicare claims for their patients, but occasionally the patient must file the claim. It is necessary to have the physician's signature on the form *or* to send in the bills, containing his signature, along with the form to the insurance company which handles Medicare in the area where the patient lives. Such a company is called the *carrier.* I tried, at first, going to the insurance office, about forty miles from where we lived, hoping to get help initially in filing claims for Mother, but no one in that office seemed interested in my problem. That does not mean, of course, that all carriers will be indifferent. Actually, I had better success with this one by mail, and a friend assures me that she has received good guidance and advice over the telephone.

Finally, by trial and error, I learned to file a claim for *everything,* if the doctor had not already done so, rather than spend hours trying to figure out what Mother was or was not entitled to. Then, when the reply came back from the Medicare carrier, I sent copies of the Medicare response and all bills to at least one, and sometimes to both, of Mother's other insurance companies. I suppose this system is somewhat unorthodox, but it worked well and I recommend it.

Now, two years after Mother's death, I have learned what I did wrong. Instead of going to the carrier, I should have gone to the Social Security office. I have done that recently to get help with filing my own claims for minor surgery, and I cannot remember ever having encountered such courtesy and helpfulness in a government office. When I admitted, with some embarrassment, that I needed help in filling out Medicare forms, the young woman I was talking to assured me that the forms are indeed complicated and that it is not unusual for people to have trouble with them. Then she explained the notice and bills I showed her, filled in the necessary parts of the Medicare claim form, and made duplicates of everything for me. Perhaps I was lucky; I have no guarantee that all helpers in Social Security offices are as courteous and helpful as the one I encountered.

One of my problems has been, and still is, knowing when I am supposed to submit the Part B Medicare form and when the physician will submit it. It would be extremely helpful if every doctor would have a sign by the reception desk, reading either "We will submit your Medicare forms" or "We do not submit Medicare forms; you must submit them yourself."

The forms seem confusing, but one learns, eventually, that only certain key spots must be filled in: name of patient, membership number, nature of illness, for example. If the doctor's bills are submitted along with the claim, his signature is not needed on the form. It is wise to keep copies of everything, as they may be needed when reporting income taxes. Medical expenses that are not paid by Medicare or other insurance are often tax deductible.

In summary I have the following suggestions for making the most of Medicare and other insurance:

1. Ask the receptionist, before leaving the doctor's office, if the *bill* will be sent to Medicare or to you.
2. If the bill is to be sent to you, ask if the *claim form* will be sent to the carrier by the doctor's office, or if you should submit it to the carrier.
3. If you must submit the claim yourself, send all bills with it, making copies for your records. Since the bills will contain the doctor's signature, he will not even need to sign the claim.

Medicare does not pay for everything. For Part A there is a $304 deductible clause, and for Part B $75 is deductible (1983). These amounts change from year to year. In 1983 the patient had to pay $304 in hospital expenses, before Medicare paid anything, and $75 in physician's bills, before Medicare paid. After deductions, Medicare pays only a certain percentage of the bills. For this reason supplementary insurance is needed.

Mother's MIA policy was supplemental insurance, which paid whatever Medicare did not pay for; that is, it paid the deductible and also whatver percent of the remainder was not covered. The Colonial Penn policy was more independent; it paid Mother's expenses, or part of them, regardless of what Medicare did or did not do. In 1970 it paid the only really large hospital bill that Mother ever had; over eight hundred dollars for all kinds of tests, including a brain scan, given her while she stayed in the hospital for a few days. Medicare did not pay for the hospital expenses, I believe because she was in the hospital not because of illness but for diagnostic tests. I did not try to use the MIA insurance.

There are some expenses which no insurance will cover. During this hospital stay Mother had to have a "sitter" with her for all but the hours between midnight and six a.m. I stayed with her a good part of the time, and her sisters, cousins, and nieces came in to spell me frequently. In the evening I paid $1.50 an hour (it would be over twice that today) to a woman who stayed with Mother from six until midnight. Although this service was necessary because of Mother's mental condition (she was not able to ring for a nurse if she needed one), this expense was not covered by any insurance as the help given Mother was considered merely custodial.

Since most insurance policies cover just about the same things, carrying more than one is considered superfluous, and I believe that if I had understood better the way in which Mother's MIA policy worked, the other policy would have been unnecessary. At present, scare tactics are being used on television and in direct-mail advertising to persuade elderly people to take out additional health insurance. As a result, some people have impoverished themselves.An article in the November 1981 *Reader's Digest*, "Beware the Medi-Scare Con Game!" by Karen E. Hunt, cites examples of elderly people who carry thirteen, seventeen, nineteen, even *ninety* health and life insurance policies. The article recommends buying one good supplemental policy rather than a number of incomplete ones. It maintains that one cannot close all the gaps by buying multiple policies and points out that a coordination of benefits clause in most policies prohibits collecting from more than one company at a time.

Neither Medicare nor other health insurance usually pays for custodial care, which is what people with dementia need. Medicare and other policies will pay for such services only under certain conditions: the patient must have been in a hospital, needing medical care, for a certain period of time preceding her stay in an extended care facility or a nursing home. Even then, the financial reimbursement is limited to a few weeks. Medicaid, however, for which people with genuine financial hardship are eligible, does pay for custodial care for an un-limited length of time.

It is possible to obtain financial aid if a person is suffering from a mental illness rather than a mental disorder. (See Chapter II, Definitions) The amount that Medicare will pay is limited: in 1982, it was $250 a year for outpatient treatment by a doctor, and no more than 190 days of care in a psychiatric hospital *in the patient's lifetime*. There are other possibilities, however: State hospitals and Veterans' Hospitals for those who qualify.

It is a comfort to know that an elderly person is entitled to Social Security, to Medicare, sometimes to Medicaid. But there is another side of the coin. When people are employed, taxes have to be paid to provide such insurance for their old age.

While Mother was living with me and we had someone staying with her, social security taxes had to be paid for that person. Every quarter I had to send a report to the federal government of how much money had been paid, with check for a specified amount, a percentage of her salary. At four hundred dollars a month (plus room and board, but fortunately the government seemed interested only in the cash outlay), that was $1200 quarterly on which the tax had to be paid on Essie's salary. Theoretically, the employee is supposed to have half the tax deducted from her salary. But I never made such an arrangement. Instead, I paid out the entire amount, using Mother's money, of course. It seemed to me at the time to be a cruel tax. We had to pay the salary so that I could work; then we had to pay a tax on the salary. Nor was the salary tax-deductible, nor would it have been even if Mother had been a dependent.

But Essie, too, is entitled to Social Security.

To be a dependent, a parent today must have an annual gross income of less than one thousand dollars a year. Tax-exempt income, such as social security payments, is not included in gross income. A single adult daughter or son caring for a parent with such a limited income could also be considered head of a household, even if the parent were in a nursing home. This would result in considerable income tax savings for the son or daughter. The amount paid for the parent's care, however, would not be tax-deductible. If a parent were considered "physically or mentally incapacitated," such expenses would be deductible, but a person with dementia, who is generally not completely helpless, would probably not qualify. Nor would custodial help at home be covered by Medicare or by co-insurance policies though it would probably be covered by Medicaid in some cases.

Dementia is an expensive disease. One can understand the logic behind the question asked by a woman who went to the Social Security office for help. "How much will the government pay me," she inquired, "if I keep my mother at home?"

My mother had done everything within reason to provide for her old age, so that she would not be financially dependent. She had bought property, she had two health insurance policies, she had a small retirement income, and she was fortunate enough to have Social Security and Medicare. She also had three life insurance policies. One was part of her state retirement package, one was a paid-up policy which she had bought when she was very young, and one was a larger policy on which she was still making payments.

Considerable money had been borrowed on each of the last two, and I was tempted, from time to time, to pay back the loans and to cash in the policies. When she died, I was glad that I had not done so as the policies could be converted into ready cash to pay her funeral expenses, whereas the rest of the estate was tied up for a few months. The interest on the loans was very low, and it would have been foolish to pay these loans off, since money invested, even in a savings account, would bring in a higher rate. Also, if cashed before her death, the policies would have been worth much less than they were worth after she died. Most important, when all other assets (her bonds, the money in her checking and savings accounts) were frozen, the life insurance money came in as soon as I requested it and submitted copies of her death certificate.

Even though mother's income was small and she seldom had to pay taxes, her income tax had to be filed each year, including the year after her death. Not only had she always filed her own taxes; for many years she had computed mine as well. Eventually I took over my own taxes, but when she became ill I did not have the courage to do hers, as simple as they were. Instead, I engaged a lawyer to take care of hers and mine. Many people prefer to use a tax consultant, but I felt more secure with a family lawyer who took care of everything: taxes, power of attorney, will, and settling her estate.

The last arrangement that needs to be taken care of is the funeral. I wish that I had talked over funeral plans with Mother while she was still able to carry on a discussion but I was embarrassed. So when she died I had only vague plans. I called her minister, who recommended a mortician who took over with great efficiency. Having read Nancy Mitford's *The American Way of Death,* I was aware that any funeral home would try to sell me the highest package, so I asked the funeral director to show me the lowest-priced coffin first. (The price of the coffin included all other, or almost all other, expenses.) I chose the second-lowest-priced one, which seemed to me simple but dignified. I did not believe that my mother would have selected, herself, an ornate and expensive coffin. In fact, she had years earlier expressed an interest in cremation, but I felt that the funeral was necessary for the benefit of her sisters, who were somewhat traditional about burial customs. The funeral director admitted that if I had not expressed a desire to see the lower-priced coffins first, she would have started with the most expensive.

I miss my mother, both as she was when she was younger and alert and as she was after she became a victim of dementia. Even then, for many years she maintained her sense of humor. Once when she was trying to select earrings to wear to church and it was already time for the service to begin, I said to her, "Mother, what is St. Peter going to say to you when you are late arriving in heaven, because you could not make up your mind which jewels to wear?"

"I guess he will just tell me to go to hell," she promptly replied.

Sometimes I even miss my visits to the nursing home, and I still occasionally go to see the patients who were there with her and who are still alive. The one thing I never miss, however, is the responsibility for her finances.

Notes to Chapter VIII

1. Anne-Marie Schiro, New York Times News Service, in Saturday *Herald and Leader,* Lexington, Kentucky, June 6, 1981, p. D 4

2. Quoted in Michael Briley, "How to Find the Right Lawyer," *Modern Maturity,* April-May, 1982, p. 6

CHAPTER IX

Recent Research

Nobody seemed to know what to do about my mother's dementia, but while she was suffering from it there were people looking for answers, and they are still looking. Although no cure for true dementia has been found, improved methods of diagnosis have been developed, making it possible to identify the pseudo-dementias, such as depression, which can often be reversed. Meanwhile, researchers continue in their efforts to identify the causes of true dementias and to search for cures. Behind this research, and basic to it, is our knowledge of the human brain, an area which has been called the "last frontier" of medical science. Our understanding of the brain and how it works has been gaining momentum since the turn of the century and has had remarkable effects on both medicine and psychology.

When I examined the nervous system of an earthworm in my college zoology class, I was amazed at the complexity of that humble creature. I am still in awe of all such phenomena, and it is with humility that I attempt to describe the much greater complexities of the human brain. The more I learn of it, the more respect I have for the scientists who have explored its intricate design and its seemingly infinite components.

It is a complex organism of billions of nerve cells, or neurons, sending messages to each other by means of neurotransmitters. Since these neurons will not regenerate, as some other cells sometimes will—in skin, for example—it is fortunate indeed that we have so many of them.[1]

A neuron resembles a fried egg with the white "splatted out into fingers."[2] The gap between neurons is called a synapse. It is across these synapses that the neurotransmitters send messages. By marking some transmitters with radioactive chemicals, then tracing them with a modified Geiger counter, scientists can observe them.

The fibers which extend from the central cell body are called axons and dendrites. They do not actually touch, but come close to each other. The axons send messages; the dendrites receive them. Most neurons have one axon and a number of dendrites. An electrical impulse travels down the axon. It manufactures and releases a neurotransmitter substance, a chemical, which goes to a dendrite of another neuron, which may send the impulse down its own axon. Or it may not. What the second neuron does depends on the incoming messages it is getting from other neurons, the total impact. At each synapse, the neurotransmitter chemicals may be reabsorbed by other neurons, or they may be chemically destroyed. All this is happening at the rate of several cycles a second in each neuron.[3] The human brain is an incredibly busy place.

It is larger than the brains of most animals, but more important, a greater proportion of it is "uncommitted" to motor, auditory, olfactory, and visual functions than is true of animals. It is because of the high percentage of uncommitted area in the cortex of their brains that human beings have a much greater capacity for activity than have the lower animals.[4]

One area of the brain, called the hippocampus, is important in memory storage. Although a normal aged brain and the brain of a dementia patient weigh about the same, the number of neurons in the hippocampus of the dementia patient is greatly reduced. Furthermore, the plaques and tangles which characterize Alzheimer's disease are especially common in the hippocampus area.[5]

The brain is divided into two hemispheres, connected by a pathway called the corpus callosum, through which they communicate with each other. In the nineteenth century a French surgeon, Paul Broca (1824-1880), discovered that the seat of articulate speech is located in the left side of the brain in most people regardless of handedness. In left-handed people the center may sometimes be in the right hemisphere. For a long time it was believed that the left cerebral hemisphere was of greater importance than the right. Later research, however, has proved the right hemisphere to be in some ways, such as spacial relationships and intuitive thinking, superior.

In 1963 Dr. Robert Sperry of the California Institute of Technology proved that epileptic seizures started in one hemisphere and were conducted across the corpus callosum to the opposite hemisphere.[6] Sperry had previously experimented on animals, severing the network of nerve fibers connecting the two hemispheres of the brain. He found that when these animals had learned a task by means of the stimulation of one hemisphere, they could still perform it after the operation, when stimulated in that hemisphere, but not when stimulated in the other. However, they could *be taught to perform similar tasks* when stimulated in the other hemisphere. When epileptics underwent similar surgery to control seizures, they suffered no obvious changes in mental ability.[7]

From my limited experience, it would seem that the specific symptoms of a dementia patient might possibly be related to the side of the brain that is more severely damaged. My mother, for example, sometimes had trouble remembering words; she also appeared to become lefthanded. Could that mean that the left side of her brain, which controlled her speech, was more affected than the right, and that the right side was compensating for it?

One of Mother's early symptoms was her reluctance to play bridge, a game at which she had excelled. Recently a man said to be in the early stages of Alzheimer's disease was shown on television. He had trouble remembering words, but he could still play bridge. If his right hemisphere was less damaged than his left, perhaps he could remember the forms and shapes of the cards. That does not explain, however, how he could remember the bidding.

There are many unanswered questions about the last ten years of my mother's life; I shall never know exactly what caused her mental confusion. An autopsy might have shown precisely what her condition was, but I did not ask for one. I wish now that I had. It is strangely disturbing to know so little about her so-called "terminal" illness. All we really know is that her mind, especially her short-term memory, was seriously affected, and that her condition was considered irreversible. Since at one time she had extensive tests, I am reasonably sure that she had a true dementia, not a pseudo-dementia.

To families of patients who appear to have senile dementia, the most meaningful research has been that which enables doctors to differentiate between true and pseudo-dementia. A recent book by Henry Edwards, *What Happened to My Mother*,[8] reveals the tragic results of confusing the two. The disturbing symptoms of Edwards' mother were the result of depression, and she was eventually cured—but only after she suffered at the hands of incompetent doctors and indifferent aides in the mental ward to which she was first sent. With a less caring and a less determined family, she no doubt would have stayed there until she died. Fortunately, her son was persistent in his search for help for her, and she was admitted to another hospital, where anti-depressant medicine was prescribed. She recovered completely and now leads a normal life.

At least two blood tests are available to help identify one type of depression, called unipolar depression. One test measures levels of hormones known to be unusually high in persons with this type of depression; the other test measures patterns of responses in hormone levels. Although not infallible, the tests, according to Dr. A. L. C. Pottash of Fair Oaks Hospital in Summit, New Jersey, have a high degree of accuracy.[9]

Since Alzheimer's disease is now known to be the most common of the dementias, recent research has tried to improve methods of identifying it. At present it can be confirmed only after death, when brain tissue can be examined microscopically. So neurologists use a process of elimination: if a patient's tests show that she is not suffering from depression, reaction to drugs, chemical imbalance, oxygen shortage caused by heart and lung problems, or some other identifiable cause, then she has one of the "true" dementias, probably Alzheimer's disease or multi-infarct dementia, sometimes called "hardening of the arteries of the brain" or "cerebral arteriosclerosis."[10]

Some true dementias can be identified easily, since other symptoms appear before dementia becomes apparent. The dementia appears in the advanced stages. Such diseases include multiple sclerosis, Huntington's disease, Pick's disease, Parkinson's disease, and Creutzfeld-Jakob disease. The cause of some of these diseases is known already. Scientists continue to look for the causes of others and of Alzheimer's disease. To help identify them and many other conditions a number of devices and tests have been developed.

Two such devices, with names much too difficult for the layman, are *computerized axial tomography* and *positron emission tomography*. They make it possible for a doctor to look into a brain and identify first, what is there, and second, what it is doing. Fortunately for those of us who are illiterate in technology, the initials of these terms form happy acronyms: CAT and PET. Another even newer device, nuclear magnetic resonance, known as NMR, may make the CAT scanner obsolete in a few years.

The CAT scanner has been around for some time. It produces X-rays which can reveal brain tumors and other disorders. But it does not reveal how well the brain with the tumor or with some less obvious abnormality is functioning or even whether it is functioning at all.

The PET scanner enables one to see metabolism in action. It provides a kind of "window" through which researchers can see what is happening. PET scanners are still in a developmental stage, but eventually they may provide solutions to many puzzles, including the cause of dementia. Their components consist of supersensitive radiation detectors, a highly sophisticated computer, a cyclotron that generates radiosotopes, and a radiochemistry laboratory. The entire process of scanning, transmitting, recording, computer analyzing, and displaying takes from five to ten minutes. The result is a "computer-processed, color-coded picture that . . . tells the physician which parts of the patient's brain are active and how active they are."[11]

Unfortunately, few hospitals can afford this miracle machine, which costs over seven million dollars. A less expensive technique, called ultra-sound, is being used in some hospitals and health centers. Although it can detect the movement of blood through a large vessel and the build-up of plaques in arteries, and thus help detect atherosclerosis, it cannot monitor the brain.

Another method which is said to be capable of testing for dementias is called neurometrics. Developed by a group of psychobiologists at the Brain Research Laboratories of New

York University Medical Center, it analyzes the electrical measurements of brain activity. Since it does not necessarily rely on verbal descriptions, but evokes responses to colors and shapes, it is free of cultural bias. It is said to be able to aid in the diagnosis both of retardation of children and of dementia in adults.[12]

It has been predicted that within the next few years neurometric terminals may be available in doctors' offices, health centers, and in schools. A telephone link-up with a central analysis center will be available in physicians' offices, information will be relayed to the center, and a computer will receive from the analysis center a printout of the diagnosis.[13]

While some researchers are developing methods of diagnosing dementia, others are attempting to find the causes, especially of Alzheimer's disease. A possible cause, it has been discovered, is a chemical deficiency in some of the patient's neurotransmitters; an enzyme called choline acetyltransferase, needed to manufacture acetylcholine, an important transmitter, is deficient in patients with Alzheimer's disease. Many neurons which use this transmitter are found in the hippocampus, the small cluster of cells important in memory.[14] A very recent finding at Johns Hopkins is reported by Gina Kolata in SCIENCE. This shows that in Alzheimer's there is a decrease of cell numbers in the nucleus basalis of Maynert which is responsible for ACH production to the brain.[15]

According to Dr. Peter Davies of the Albert Einstein College of Medicine in New York, this chemical deficiency is much greater in Alzheimer's patients than in the brains of other elderly people. Although a person of ninety or ninety-five will probably have only thirty percent of the amount of the enzyme he had as a young adult, he will not suffer noticeably from this decline. On the other hand, an Alzheimer's patient of sixty or seventy will have only ten percent of the adult level of the enzyme. It is believed that the level can drop to twenty percent of the young adult level without harm. The next five percent, however, will probably cause serious trouble.[16]

These neurochemical changes are one possible cause of Alzheimer's disease. Others are metal deposits, genetic factors, infectious agents, and immunological defects.[17]

Metal deposits, especially of aluminum and manganese, have been found in Alzheimer's patients. Furthermore, when aluminum was injected into animals they developed the tangles and plaques typical of Alzheimer's disease. But aluminum levels increase with age, according to some researchers, regardless of the presence or absence of this dementia; and even the experiments with animals are not conclusive evidence.

A long-range study on the island of Guam, where the native Chamorro Indians are highly susceptible to several brain diseases, should be enlightening. A number of dementia patients there are being examined periodically, and after their death their symptoms are to be correlated with changes in their brains. At the same time, tissue from the Guamanians who die from other diseases will also be examined. One purpose of this study is to determine the normal levels of trace elements throughout life and to discover whether the levels go up as a consequence of normal aging.[18]

Another possible cause of Alzheimer's disease is a defect in the body's immunological system. This is a system whereby bacteria are attacked and destroyed. Sometimes, however, possibly as a result of aging, the immune system attacks the body's own tissue. If this tissue consists of brain cells, scavenger cells seek out the brain neurons and destroy them. The abnormal plaque material that results may then accumulate outside the cells, "like so much trash in corridors." [19]

There is some evidence that Alzheimer's disease results from a slow virus infection. Two researchers in Bethesda, Maryland, Dr. D. Carleton Gajdusek and Dr. Clarence J. Gibbs, Jr., have discovered that two other brain diseases, kuru and Creutzfeldt-Jakob disease, are caused by a slow-acting virus. These scientists have injected extracts from the brains of Alzheimer's disease patients into the brains of chimpanzees, which developed signs of dementia after a period of two months. Another experiment involved putting extracts from the brains of Alzheimer's patients into laboratory cultures of fetal human brain cells. The changes that took place resembled those seen in the persons who died of Alzheimer's.[20]

Although both of these experiments seem impressive to the layman, the results are not considered, even by scientists who worked on them, to be conclusive. They have apparently been convincing enough to frighten some pathologists, however, who have reportedly refused to perform autopsies on suspected Alzheimer and Creutzfeldt-Jakob patients for fear that they will be infected.[21]

More disturbing to the people who are related to Alzheimer's disease patients than the virus infection theory is the possibility that the disease is hereditary. No one seems to believe that heredity plays an important part, but it has been observed that people are more likely to have this disease if they have relatives who have had it. These observations have no doubt been based on some kind of statistics, which are often suspect, as anyone knows who has read a book by Darrell Huff called *How to Lie with Statistics*. I am by no means certain that my mother had Alzheimer's disease. Her illness was never diagnosed as that. She was said to have cerebral arteriosclerosis. This may have developed into multi-infarct dementia which, I understand, is caused by a series of small strokes. (An *infarct* is the death of tissue resulting from interference with its blood supply.)

If, however, what she had was Alzheimer's disease, I cannot believe that it "runs in our family." Two of her sisters behaved somewhat abnormally for a few months before they died, but I attribute their behavior to the effect of medication they were taking. One of Mother's cousins observed that people seem to have a harder time dying nowadays than they used to. Her mother, my mother's mother, and my other great-aunts lived to be well into their eighties. As they approached old age they sat in their rockers, as my cousin observed, and read their Bibles. They died quietly, often at home in bed.

Come to think of it, perhaps it was their Bible and their rockers which kept them contented and mentally healthy. A fascinating book by S. I. McMillen, *None of These Diseases*,[21] puts forth the thesis that both the Old Testament and the New Testament contain excellent advice for a long and healthy life. The specific suggestions McMillen enumerates range from taking sanitary precautions to turning the other cheek.

Even if a Bible and a rocking chair cannot prevent dementia (and I am not seriously suggesting that they can), they seem to add to the patient's comfort and contentment. Mrs. S., Mother's roommate who always held her Bible on her lap, was among the calmest of patients. And Mother herself was never more contented, when she lived with me, than when she sat in a rockingchair holding her infant great-grandson, David.

Notes to Chapter IX

1. Steven Rose, *The Conscious Brain*. New York: Alfred Knopf, 1973. p. 148

2. Adam Smith, *Powers of the Mind*. New York: Random House, 1975. p. 142

3. Morton Hunt, *The Universe Within: A New Science Explores the Human Mind*. New York: Simon and Schuster, 1982. p. 41 ff.

4. *Ibid.*, p. 36

5. Lawrence Galton, *The Truth About Senility*. New York: Crowell, 1979. pp. 24-25

6. Richard Restak, *The Brain: The Last Frontier*. Garden City, New York: Doubleday and Co., 1979. p. 171

7. "Medicine: Three Pioneers of the Brain," *Time*, October 19, 1981. p. 95

8. Henry Edwards, *What Happened to My Mother*. New York: Harper and Row, 1982.

9. "Medifacts," *Woman's Day*, September 1, 1981. p. 8

10. U.S. Department of Health and Human Services, *The Dementias: Hope Through Research*. 1981, pp. 8-12

11. Alcestis Oberg and Daniel Woodard, "Anti-Matter Mind Probes and Other Medical Miracles," *Science Digest*, April 1982.

12. Restak, pp. 268-277

13. *Ibid.*

14. *The Dementias*, p. 16

15. Gina Kolata. *Clues to Alzheimer's Disease Emerge. Science*, February, 1983

16. Harold M. Schmeck, Jr. "Research Attempts to Fight Senility." The New York *Times*, July 31, 1979

17. *The Dementias*, pp. 17-20

18. *Ibid.*
19. *Ibid.*
20. Schmeck.
21. Richard Trubo, "The Senility Virus." *Science Digest,* August 1981. p. 124
22. S. I. McMillen, M.D., *None of These Diseases.* Old Tappan, New Jersey: Spire Books, 1963

CHAPTER X

Cures and Prevention: Some Possibilities

Along with the search for causes, experiments to determine the most effective treatment for dementia are constantly being conducted. Some of the possible cures involve the use of drugs; some involve surgery; some involve both. Possible preventive measures include inoculation, diet, and exercise. The symptoms in people who have already contracted a form of dementia may be reversed, perhaps, or at least kept from getting worse, or slowed down somewhat, by such means as diet and exercise or by reality orientation and other forms of psychiatric therapy.

Probably the most conventional treatment for senile dementia is the use of drugs to expand blood vessels, so that they can carry more blood to the brain. Such drugs are called vasodilators. According to Lawrence Galton, some relief of confusion and improvement in mental alertness and memory have resulted from their use.[1]

Though some patients have reportedly benefited from these drugs, becoming less confused and more alert, the benefits have not always correlated with increased blood flow. Dilation, therefore, may not be the major effect of some vasodilators. Some may improve the brain's use of oxygen and nutrients, and some perhaps help restore the proper chemical balance.[2]

A drug called physostigmine (why do all drugs have unpronounceable names?) keeps acetylcholine from rapidly breaking down after it is released from nerve cells. There is some evidence that this drug helps, but there are unpleasant side effects.[3]

Dr. David de Wied, in the Netherlands, has found that vasopressin, a pituitary hormone, affects memory.[4] This drug is being tested on patients at the National Institute of Health Clinical Center in Bethesda, Maryland. It is given as an inhalant, as there is evidence that nerve endings which are sensitive to smell may pick it up and carry it to the brain/The Dutch investigators have used it in experiments involving rats. If they made a wrong turn in a simple T-shaped maze, the rats were given a mild electric shock. When they were given injections of vasopressin, either before or shortly after they explored the maze, their memories improved. When they were retested up to 48 or 72 hours after the first trial, many of the rats treated with vasopressin avoided the shock, while the untreated rats usually forgot which side of the maze was associated with the shock after 24 hours.[5]

According to Dr. Jerome Yesavage of the Stanford Medical School, about twenty percent of patients who were given a drug called dihydroergotozine mesylate (sold as Hydergine), showed some improvement. It is said to work better in preventing mild dementia from getting worse than in more advanced cases. Not all doctors will prescribe this drug, but Dr. Yesavage maintains that he would take it himself, if he had Alzheimer's.[6]

Drugs that bind aluminum, to eliminate that metal from the blood, are being tried at the Ohio State University.[7]

A "memory pill" containing lecithin, a substance commonly found in many foods, once showed promise of producing a revival of memory in dementia patients, but a report in the Journal of Gerontology maintains that the drug is ineffective.[8] Researchers at Tufts University have tried feeding pure lecithin to senile patients and to healthy ones, to see if memory improved, but so far the improvement has not been marked.

Patients with Parkinson's disease have been treated successfully with L-dopa, a drug which is converted in the body into a neurotransmitter. According to Galton, it is possible that the same drug may be used to help patients with other forms of dementia, but the results of research in this area indicate that it will be a long time before failing mental powers can be restored by this treatment.

Before L-dopa was introduced as a treatment for Parkinson's disease, a young surgeon, Dr. Irving S. Cooper, demonstrated that Parkinson's could be successfully controlled by brain surgery. He cured many cases, reversing by skillful surgery the involuntary movement disorders that accompany this disease. His autobiography, entitled *The Vital Probe: My Life as a Brain Surgeon,*[9] is both informative and readable. Perhaps some day a surgeon will discover a way to reverse senile dementia by surgery.

A few years ago a neuro-surgeon at Johns Hopkins operated on a sixty-year-old woman who was suffering from little strokes. After removing a piece of bone from the back of her skull, he lifted an atherosclerotic plaque from an artery; the plaque was preventing an adequate blood supply from reaching the brain. This microsurgery took 10½ hours. The operation was risky, but successful, and the woman was greatly relieved, as it removed the possibility that she would have a massive stroke. "I would rather have died under the surgery," she said, "than have lived to be a vegetable."[10]

Surgeons in Stockholm, in 1981, were planning to transplant tissue into the brain of a patient with Parkinson's disease, the first attempt at such an operation. The cells were to be taken from the patient's own adrenal glands, and to be implanted in his brain in the hope of stopping the tremors that are typical of Parkinson's. Eight years of research and animal experiments at the National Institute of Mental Health in Washington, D.C., and at the University of Colorado Health Sciences Center in Denver had preceded the operation on humans. The tests on animals have shown that the brain does not reject transplants, as other parts of the body do. The Americans were not planning to participate in the operation on a human patient, who was to be one who had not responded to conventional treatment with L-dopa.[11]

A recent "wonder tool" of medicine is the laser beam, which can select its target and can be used almost any place in the body. At the Erie County Medical Center in Buffalo, New York, it has been used to vaporize brain tumors.[12]

A small company in Maryland holds a patent on the "biochip," a device which operates in the same manner as the chips in a computer, but is designed for use in the human body. In the future these biochips may be used to channel electrical impulses and bridge a severed spinal cord, thus helping a patient to regain his ability to walk. Or they may be used to restore sight, or to detect and regulate improper rhythms in an elderly patient's heart. Researchers intend to implant the chips in animals before attempting to use them in humans. Real advances are not expected for four or five years.[13]

If all this is possible, it may be reasonable to hope that in the future the biochip will be used in some way to reverse the symptoms of dementia.

Until such time as biochips, or drugs, or surgery, can reverse the dementias which are now irreversible, there is some help, for families as well as patients, in group therapy. The Burke Rehabilitation Center for Alzheimer's Disease and Related Disorders provides psychiatric help and counseling for patients and their families. This Center and others like it perform an invaluable service.

They have arisen in part at least because of the tireless work of Bobbie Glaze, whose husband became a victim of Alzheimer's disease in 1970. At that time she was given the following diagnosis:

> Your husband has Alzheimer's disease, a progressive, irreversible brain deterioration, for which there is no known cause or treatment.

When her husband became violent, even nursing homes would not keep him. Finally he was admitted to a Veteran's Administration hospital. Mrs. Glaze, as a result of her husband's illness, started a support group for families with dementing illnesses. In 1979 seven such groups united to form the Alzheimer's Disease and Related Disorders Association, with headquarters now located at 360 N. Michigan Avenue, Room 601, Chicago, Illinois 60601. It is a fast-growing organization, with affiliates spread over a wide-reaching area.

Dr. James Haycox, head of Burke's psychiatry department, has conducted intensive seven-hour programs there focusing on memory training and group therapy. He believes that the program helped to slow down the disease, or at least the symptoms. The cost was $53.00 a day, and patients were not reimbursed by Medicare, since it considers the rehabilitation of Alzheimer's patients impossible.[14]

As early as 1958 a young psychiatrist, James C. Folsom, began a program called Reality Orientation. The technique seems simple. The patient is reminded frequently of who he is, who the speaker is, what day it is, what time it is, and when the next meal will be served. Sometimes a class is held, in which members are drilled in their names, the names of others, the date, and sometimes more difficult matters. To succeed, Reality Orientation is supposed to be a twenty-four-hour-a-day affair. Folsom, who started the program at the Veteran's Administration in Topeka and later introduced it at the Veteran's Hospital in Tuscaloosa, Alabama, never claimed that it would retrieve the lost parts of the brain, but he seemed to have considerable success in saving the parts of a patient's brain that were still functioning. In other words, the method will not reverse dementia, but perhaps to a certain extent it arrests it. According to Dr. Miriam Aronson, psychiatrist at Albert Einstein Medical School, the goal is to "maintain the disoriented at a level of disorientation which may be less than if you ignored them."[15]

In addition to Reality Orientation and other therapy programs, attempts are being made to reverse or at least arrest dementia symptoms through diet. Patients have been given food containing large amounts of material that makes up acetylcholine, but the results have been inconclusive. Since cholesterol is found in atherosclerotic deposits, it is considered a wise precaution to avoid too much of it in the diet. It is found in meat, dairy products, eggs, and organ meats. A diet emphasizing vegetables, cereals, fish, and little meat is recommended. Hot dogs and potato chips, both loaded with saturated fats, should especially be avoided.[16]

Often relatives of Alzheimer's patients are concerned that they, too, may develop the disease, and wonder how it can be prevented. Since the cause is not known, no one can be sure of the prevention. But then, that is true of all diseases. Although the chances of contracting lung cancer are reduced by not smoking, there is no guarantee that a non-smoker will not get that disease.

The sensible approach, especially for people who are past middle-age, is to pay particular attention to diet and exercise, and hope for the best.

Whether my mother's diet had anything to do with her

having dementia I do not know. For the most part she ate sensibly: a moderate amount of meat (she preferred chicken or fish); fresh vegetables, not overcooked; green salads; fruit of all kinds. But she did eat an unusually large amount of butter. She used to make the most delicious rolls that I have ever eaten. The recipe called for a great deal of butter, and she brushed them with butter just before putting them in the oven. I never understood why, but when she ate one she would add *more* butter to it. She also put extra butter on mashed potatoes, whether it was needed or not, and on toast which had already been buttered.

Exercise may be as important as diet. Dr. Peter D. Wood and other researchers at Stanford University kept track of a group of active men who ran fifteen miles a week, and compared their cholesterol level with that of other men of approximately the same age. The runners had only slightly less cholesterol than the others. But there are two types of cholesterol, called high density lipoproteins (HDL) and low density lipoproteins (LDL). LDL carries cholesterol to the tissues, depositing it in artery walls, where it interferes with circulation. HDL does just the opposite. The runners had a much higher level of HDL than the nonrunners. This is considered more significant than the level of cholesterol; it showed that the runners did indeed benefit from the exercise.[17]

Dr. Kenneth Cooper, who has worked with officers and recruits at Maxwell Air Force Base in Alabama, at Lackland Air Force Base in Texas, and with astronauts at the Space Systems Division in Los Angeles, is an exercise specialist with missionary zeal. In addition to building up healthy bodies, according to Dr. Cooper, the people he worked with "gained the ability to relax, were less anxious, had a better self-image and more confidence in themselves."[18]

After the age of about fifty my mother took hardly any exercise. When she was younger she swam occasionally, and at one time she rode horseback fairly regularly with a friend who owned horses and needed to exercise them. But I never knew her to take any kind of exercise for the sake of her health, or just because she enjoyed it. For her, it was another form of socializing; if she had friends who swam, she swam with them, and if someone invited her to go horseback riding, she went.

When she stayed with me she liked to walk to the corner of our street and back, especially if I went with her. That was not exactly exercise, however, as she moved so slowly that it was tiring for me to move along with her. When she first went to the Extended Care Unit I tried taking her for walks, but when she returned to her room she seemed more disoriented than ever, so I gave up the idea. I often found her walking up and down the corridor, holding on to a railing, but she looked lost and pathetic.

When I had to put Mother in a nursing home, I was sorry that I could not find one with a pool and a supervised swimming program. As far as I know, no such home exists. Water itself is therapeutic, and it would not seem to be asking too much to have a warm shallow pool available for patients, though I realize that such a luxury would necessarily increase the cost of the home considerably. But for many patients it would be worth it.

In the last few years a special exercise program for adults, called Body Recall, has been developed by Dorothy Chrisman, a physical education instructor at Berea College in Kentucky. Mrs. Chrisman travels around the country with a team of five or six men and women, whose average age is seventy-two, demonstrating the kinds of exercises suitable for older people. The team has given demonstrations in nursing homes and veterans' hospitals, always with audience participation.[19]

Some of her students have found the exercises stimulating mentally as well as physically. One woman who was attending the class was diagnosed as having Alzheimer's disease. According to her daughter, after each class session she was more alert than usual, exhibiting very little evidence of disorientation.

Along with exercise and proper nutrition, good health can be supported by mental attitude. Some people expect to be sick when they become old, and it is possible that their expectations are self-fulfilling. Actually, people over sixty-five have fewer acute illnesses than younger people, though they may acquire chronic conditions and suffer some loss of hearing or sight. But these problems need not keep them from being active.

Musicians, especially symphony orchestra directors, live

longer than most people and continue to enjoy their work until an advanced age. Perhaps this is because conducting an orchestra requires both physical movement and mental alertness.

Today there are all sorts of opportunities for older people to renew skills they developed when younger and even to acquire new ones. There are elderhostel programs at colleges and universities; there are senior citizen centers; there are special camps for older people. The opportunities are virtually unlimited.

Better yet, there are opportunities to do volunteer work, or even work with pay sometimes, as "foster grandparents" to children in institutions. Nothing, I believe, keeps one healthier than living around children.

Perhaps I am overly optimistic, but I believe that within a few years at least some forms of dementia will be better understood and that there is a good chance they will disappear. Meanwhile, let us sincerely hope

. . . that people with pseudo-dementias will be correctly diagnosed;

. . . that people with true dementias will spend their last years in comfort and at least a measure of peace and contentment;

. . . that the owners and managers of nursing homes will find better ways of keeping patients contented, without relying too heavily on drugs;

. . . that nurses and nurses' aides will have the patience and good will required to take care of people who cannot care for themselves;

. . . that neurosurgeons will continue their miraculous operations;

. . . that researchers will find the cause or causes of Alzheimer's disease;

. . . that doctors will find ways of preventing this disease and a way to cure it.

Notes to Chapter X

1. Lawrence Galton, *The Truth About Senility.* New York: Crowell, 1979. p. 214

2. *Ibid.*

3. U.S. Department of Health and Human Services, *The Dementias: Hope Through Research,* 1981, p. 21

4. Galton, pp. 214-215

5. *The Dementias,* p. 21

6. "Your Body and Mind as the Years Go By," *Changing Times,* April 1982, pp. 54-57

7. *The Dementias,* p. 22

8. *Lecithin and Memory in Suspected Alzheimer's Disease,* Journal of Gerontology, 37, 1, January 19, 1982, pp. 4-9

9. Irving S. Cooper, *The Vital Probe: My Life as a Brain Surgeon.* New York: W. W. Norton, 1981

10. Victor Cohn in Washington *Post,* quoted in *Reader's Digest,* May 1981, pp. 55-56

11. Walter Sullivan, New York Times News Service, "Parkinson's Disease Patient to Get Brain Implant," in Lexington *Herald-Leader,* November 26, 1981, E13

12. Stanley L. Englebardt, "Lasers: Medicine's Ray of Hope," *Reader's Digest,* January 1981, pp. 169-176

13. Steve Sternberg, Knight-Ridder News Service. "Chips Could Make 'bionic' Man a Reality," Lexington *Herald,* March 3, 1982

14. Tessa Melvin, "New Center Fights Big Killer of the Aged," New York *Times,* December 6, 1981, XXII, 1:1

15. Dr. Arthur S. Freese, *The End of Senility.* New York: Arbor House, 1978. p. 156

16. Galton, pp. 197-198

17. Galton, pp. 198-199

18. William Hoffman and Jerry Shields, *Doctors on the New Frontier.* New York: Macmillan Publishing Co., Inc. p. 52

19. Dorothy Chrisman, *Body Recall: A Program of Physical Fitness for the Adult.* Berea, Kentucky: the Berea College Press, 1980. p. 1.

Some Helpful Reading

A. MAGAZINE ARTICLES

Adler, Jerry with Deborah Witherspoon. "New Looks Inside the Body." *Newsweek,* August 16, 1982. Describes new methods of diagnosis, including the use of PET scanning, CAT scanning, and ultrasound.

Alexander, Tom. "The New Technology of the Mind." *Fortune,* January 24, 1983. Summarizes and evaluates recent research in psychobiology; discusses drugs used to treat both physiological and psychosomatic diseases.

Begley, Sharon et al. "How the Brain Works." *Newsweek,* February 7, 1983. Explores the complexity of the brain and summarizes recent research in neuroscience.

Clark, Matt et al. "The Scourge of Senility." *Newsweek,* September 15, 1980. Emphasizes the symptoms of Alzheimer's disease, the importance of accurate diagnosis, and methods of coping with patients.

Fried, John J. "Neurotransmitters—Messengers of the Brain." *The Reader's Digest,* December 1976. Explains what neurotransmitters do; summarizes and evaluates recent research.

Kety, Seymour S. "Disorders of the Human Brain." *Scientific American,* September 1979. Most relevant, to people concerned with dementia, of the eleven articles about the brain contained in this issue, which have been published as a book, *The Brain,* by W. H. Freeman and Company, San Francisco.

Morris, Magdalene and Martha Rhodes. "Guidelines for the Care of Confused Patients." *American Journal of Nursing,* September 1972. Explains the difference between functional and organic confusion.

Santini, Rosemary and Katherine Barrett. "The Tragedy of Rita Hayworth." *Ladies' Home Journal,* January 1983. An interview with Rita Hayworth's daughter Yasmin

117

Khan, who describes her mother's symptoms, the early mistaken diagnosis, and the effects of her illness, more recently diagnosed as Alzheimer's disease.

Tanne, Janice Hopkins. "Alzheimer's & Aluminum: An Element of Suspicion." *American Health,* September/October 1983. Maintains that evidence of a link between aluminum and Alzheimer's disease is increasing.

Trubo, Richard. "The Senility Virus." *Science Digest,* August 1981. Demonstrates the similarity between Alzheimer's disease and Creutzfeldt-Jakob's disease and considers the possibility that the former, like the latter, is caused by a virus.

Wallis, Claudia. "Slow, Steady and Heartbreaking." *Time,* July 11, 1983. Discusses the nature of Alzheimer's disease, its possible causes, the damage to the nucleus basalis, attempted treatment with chemicals, and ways of improving the patients' quality of life.

B. BOOKS

Fox, Nancy. *You, Your Parent, and the Nursing Home.* Bend, Oregon: Geriatric Press, 1982. Contains advice on selecting a nursing home, visiting, monitoring the patient's care, dealing with doctors, evaluating the staff, being aware of the patient's medication; describes both good and bad practices in nursing homes.

Harrington, Geri. *The Medicare Answer Book.* New York: Harper & Row, 1982. Explains what Medicare does and how to use it for maximum benefits; includes chapters on supplemental policies and Health Maintenance Organizations, and a useful glossary of "medispeak."

Henig, Robin Marantz. *The Myth of Senility: Misconceptions About the Brain and Aging.* Garden City, New York: Anchor Press/Doubleday, 1981. Discusses normal aging, pseudosenility, and Alzheimer's disease; includes valuable warnings concerning self-help treatment with dietary supplements such as lecithin and vitamin E; stresses the importance of environment.

Lincoln, Elizabeth M. *Choosing a Nursing Home for the Person With Intellectual Loss.* 1980. A fourteen-page pamphlet which can be ordered from The Burke Rehabilitation Center, 785 Mamaroneck Avenue, White Plains, New York 10605.

————. *Managing the Person with Intellectual Loss (Dementia or Alzheimer's Disease) at Home.* 1980. A twelve-page manual which can be ordered from The Burke Rehabilitation Center, 785 Mamaroneck Avenue, White Plains, New York 10605.

Mace, Nancy L. and Peter V. Rabins, M.D. *The 36-Hour Day: A Family Guide to Caring for Persons with Alzheimer's Disease, Related Dementing Illnesses, and Memory Loss in Later Life.* Makes valuable suggestions for handling such diverse problems as diet, exercise, medication, behavior, outside help, financial and legal issues, nursing homes.

Reisberg, Barry, M.D. *Brain Failure: An Introduction to Concepts of Senility.* New York: The Free Press, 1981. Covers a wide range of topics, including possible causes of Alzheimer's disease and other dementias; research on prevention and treatment; and professional counseling for patients and their families.

Thornton, Susan M. and Virginia Fraser. *Understanding "Senility"—A Layperson's Guide.* Buffalo, New York: Potentials Development for Health & Aging Services, Inc., 1982. Contains helpful suggestions for caring for patients with dementia, both at home and in nursing homes.

U.S. Department of Health and Human Services. *Q & A: Alzheimer's Disease.* 1981. NIH Publication No. 80-1646. A small pamphlet which can be ordered form NIA Information Center, Room 5C-36, National Institute of Health, Bethesda, Maryland 20205.

————. *The Dementias: Hope Through Research.* A thirty-one page pamphlet which can be ordered from the NINCDS

Office of Scientific and Health Reports, HIH, Building 31, Room 8A-07, Bethesda, Maryland 20205

Waller, Ken. *How to Recover Your Medical Expenses: A Comprehensive Guide to Understanding and Unscrambling Medicare.* New York: Macmillan, 1981. Contains clear explanations and directions for using Medicare benefits; useful for anyone who is on Medicare or taking care of someone else who is.